Praise for *The Incredible Brain*

"*The Incredible Brain* is one of the most powerful, practical books I've read on living with purpose and longevity. As someone who's deeply committed to intentional living and investing in your greatest asset—yourself—this book truly hits home.

Dr. Ryan Williamson does an incredible job blending heart and science. This isn't just theory or medical jargon— He makes the science easy to understand and even easier to apply, tying it back to what matters most: your legacy, your mindset, and the daily choices that shape your life. If you're ready to live longer, feel better, and make a bigger impact in the world, *The Incredible Brain* is your roadmap."

—**Justin Donald, #1 *WSJ* and *USA Today* Best-Selling Author, Founder of The Lifestyle Investor, and Host of The Lifestyle Investor Podcast"**

"Benjamin Franklin said, "An ounce of prevention is worth a pound of cure." When it comes to health, few people and their insurance companies are willing to pay for that prevention (with either money or effort), which is unfortunate, because it is often dramatically cheaper than treating the subsequent diseases, if they can be treated at all. Thus we have a "disease care system" rather than a "health care system." We all want a long life with compressed morbidity. That is to say, we want to be healthy for our entire lives until the very end. Nobody wants ten years of dementia before they pass. Nobody wants to be disabled for decades. Real health care, i.e. prevention, doesn't just give you more years, it makes the years you have better. Following Dr. Williamson's advice in this book will teach you how to delay and even completely avoid many health conditions you never want to have. Prevention is often simple, but rarely easy. Use this guide to help make it as easy as possible."

—**James M. Dahle, MD, Emergency Physician, Best Selling Author, and Founder of The White Coat Investor**

"In a world where preventative care seems to be an afterthought, *The Incredible Brain* offers a refreshing, evidence-based guide to living not just longer, but a more impactful life. With a rare blend of scientific insight, practical strategies, and deep human wisdom, *The Incredible Brain* empowers readers to craft their own unique framework, discover their "Why", and lead lives of lasting purpose. A must-read for anyone who wants to extend their vitality and thrive -not just survive- in the years ahead."

—**Chris Board, NFL Linebacker, New York Giants**

"Accomplishing difficult tasks, such as tax planning or wealth creation, requires a strong desire and commitment. Dr. Ryan Williamson's book, *The Incredible Brain*, outlines just how a strong purpose can help you accomplish those difficult tasks."

—**Tom Wheelwright, CPA, #1 Best-selling author of** *Tax-Free Wealth*, **Founder and CEO of WealthAbility**

"*The Incredible Brain* is the perfect hybrid between actionable simplicity and scientific backup. After reading it, I feel that I now have the tools to live a longer, healthier life, giving me the ability to create a greater impact on the world."

—**Tom Burns, MD, #1 Best Selling Author of "Why Doctors Don't Get Rich", Orthopedic Surgeon, and former US Ski Team Physician**

"An absolutely compelling read. Dr. Williamson does a masterful job of providing his readers the tools on how to live purposefully and take control of their health. Speaking from experience as a former patient, Dr. Williamson takes a whole-body approach to medicine, seeking to understand the interconnectedness of all aspects of his patients' health. Using some of the latest research and data, Dr. Williamson compiles a menu of options on how to live longer with a healthy brain, body and mind."

—**Denise M. Mull, Colonel, USMC Retired**

"It is more important to know the patient that has the disease than it is to know the disease the patient has" - Sir William Osler

When I graduated from medical school in 1975, I felt like the focus at that time was disease-based medicine. There was much more emphasis on making the right diagnosis than there was on preventive approaches to treating patients. The "interesting patient" was the "enlarged liver" in room 1, the thyroid nodule in Room 6, or the "Fever of unknown origin" in Room 12. Perhaps that's why I chose to be a family physician because I enjoyed getting to know patients and having a relationship with them over time.

In the last 25 years there has been a revolution in medical education in medical schools with earlier exposure to simulated or actual clinical patients, more integration of basic and clinical science concepts throughout the curriculum, and more focus on "patient centered care", emphasizing patient autonomy, collaboration, and respect for individual preferences. The Florida State University College of Medicine, founded in 2000, was the first new medical school created in the US since the late 1970's. It was founded to address a looming physician shortage, most acute in rural and underserved areas, and met resistance from organized medicine (AMA and AAMC) that felt that we had enough doctors. FSU's vision was validated by the year 2007, when there was a call for a significant increase in medical graduates and led to a boom in creating over 30 new medical schools since that time. FSU further defied the conventional wisdom by training their graduates in community physician offices and hospitals, with the hope to encourage the graduates to practice in those communities in the future outside of the traditional specialty dominated acute care focused academic medical center.

Dr. Ryan Williamson is a 2014 graduate of the FSU College of Medicine and learned the lessons of patient focused care both at FSU and in his superb career as a neurologist in the US Navy. Caring for military service members, their families, and military retirees, he recognized that his many encounters with patients at critical end points in their lives left him asking what else could be done to live longer, healthier, and better lives. While helping patients when they were critically sick was his calling, he knew that this disease-based model was not enough. In his book, *The Incredible Brain*, he asks the reader to go beyond traditional medicine to find their purpose, take an active role in their health, and live better, healthier lives. He encourages all to develop an intentional lifestyle that is focused on optimizing sleep, nutrition, mental wellness, and physical movement. Our disease focused system does not encourage individuals to take control of their lives, harness the full power of their brain and body, and avoid the fate of those who succumb to chronic disease.

This book can serve as a handbook on how to optimize health, whether you are in your thirties or facing retirement. It provides an education on the "how" your brain and body work, and then provides practical interventions to slow the rate of aging. Each chapter is written to stand alone, providing first education that analyzes the importance of the topic for wellness, then provides "key takeaways" and a "cheat sheet" to help move the reader to better behaviors on the road to better health. I am very proud to endorse Dr. Williamson's book as a fundamental guide to prevention and self-care for all."

—John P. Fogarty, MD
Col (ret.) Medical Corps, US Army
Dean Emeritus, FSU College of Medicine

"For anyone who wants to focus on brain health and reduce their risk of poor brain outcomes, this is the read for you. Dr. Williamson does an outstanding job of discussing in a simple manner why focusing on taking care of your entire self can lead to better outcomes and a more meaningful future. He infuses his real-life experiences alongside his training and practice experience to bring to light guidance through the book. A recommended read to all looking for a healthier future."

—Jessica Ailani, MD, FAHS, Director of Georgetown
Headache Center, Professor of Clinical Neurology
Medstar Georgetown University Hospital

"Einstein said "Everything should be made as simple as possible, but not simpler."

The future of healthcare is turning towards prevention to preserve health rather than attempting to fix problems later in their course.

Dr Williamson has taken a very important topic BRAIN HEALTH and made this very complex goal simple enough for the reader to start this important process."

—**Andrew Blumenfeld, MD, Board-Certified Neurologist, Fellow of the American Academy of Neurology and American Headache Society**

"As a high-performing CEO with an APO E4/E4 diagnosis (~10x increased risk of Alzheimer's) and concussion history, my brain *is* my most valuable asset and must be protected at all costs. There is no one I trust more to advise and coach me than Dr. Ryan Williamson. Unlike countless others selling miracle cures, Ryan delivers rigorous, evidence-based research in *The Incredible Brain*. He masterfully explains complex mechanisms like neuroinflammation, then provides practical interventions you can implement immediately. His protocols have been a real life-saver. As he writes, 'You have more control than you think,' this book proves it. I believe this is essential reading for anyone serious about cognitive longevity."

—**Amber Vilhauer, Award-winning CEO of NGNG Enterprises and multi-bestselling author**

"*The Incredible Brain* is more than a book—it's a wake-up call wrapped in wisdom and rooted in science. Dr. Ryan Williamson masterfully weaves his personal story with powerful data to deliver a deeply human approach to longevity. He reminds us that living longer isn't about resisting death—it's about fully choosing life. This book invites you to reclaim your health, your purpose, and your legacy—not someday, but now. A must-read for anyone ready to become an active participant in their own vitality."

—**Nancy Levin, bestselling author of *The Art of Change* and Founder of Levin Life Coach Academy**

THE INCREDIBLE BRAIN

Proven Science Behind Living a
Longer, Healthier, More Impactful Life

THE
INCREDIBLE
BRAIN

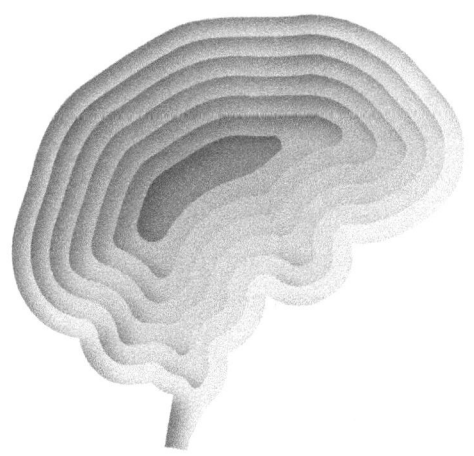

Ryan Williamson, MD

Transcend Health
Tampa, FL
Copyright © 2025 by Copyright Holder. All rights reserved.

Cataloging-in-Publication Data is on file with the Library of Congress

Paperback ISBN: 979-8-9990566-2-7
eBook ISBN: 979-8-9990566-0-3
Hardcover ISBN: 979-8-9990566-1-0

All rights reserved. No part of this publication may be reproduced, stored in a retrieval system or transmitted in any form or by any means (electronic, mechanical, photocopying, recording, or otherwise) without the written permission of the author and publisher.

Book cover and interior design by *the*BookDesigners
Editorial production by KN Literary Arts

www.transcendhealthgroup.com

Printed in the United States of America

For Tanner, my brother.

You really were the light the world so deeply needs.

Your legacy lives on.

CONTENTS

Introduction 1

1. Find Your Why 13

PART 1 — THE MECHANISMS 37
2. The Brain 39
3. The Primary Threats 75
4. The Hallmarks of Aging 125

PART 2 — THE INTERVENTIONS 163
5. Exercise 165
6. Nutrition 195
7. Sleep 235
8. Hormesis and Stress Management 265
9. Supplements 295
10. Technology 317

Conclusion 345

DISCLAIMER

In my career as a neurologist, I have treated thousands of patients. However, I am not your personal physician. I offer the information in this book for educational purposes only, not as medical advice. The content is based on scientific evidence and my professional experience, but it should not replace consultation with your personal physician. Regardless of your health status, you should consult your doctor before making any lifestyle changes based on what you read here.

The various approaches to longevity and health optimization in this book represent options to explore, not directives to follow. The decision to implement any intervention should ultimately be yours, made in consultation with medical professionals familiar with your health history.

I've also included many stories from patients of mine to illustrate how these conditions, mechanisms, and interventions apply to the real world. While these stories are true, the names of my patients have been anonymized to protect their privacy.

INTRODUCTION

THE FIFTH STROKE patient of the day had just been wheeled into the emergency department, and once again, there wasn't a single thing I could do. Unable to walk, talk, or move half of his body, he had simply arrived too late. With my head hung low, I trudged out to meet his family in the waiting room, watching their hopeful smiles fade as I explained that their dad was beyond the window for any effective intervention.

Hours later, I found myself in the cardiac ICU, consulting on the case of another gentleman who had suffered a massive heart attack earlier in the week. Six family members greeted me with the same eager gazes, and once more, I delivered the devastating news that their loved one had suffered catastrophic neurological damage and would likely never regain consciousness.

These moments—repeated countless times throughout my career as a neurologist—echo the experiences that first drew me to healthcare. One of my earliest memories is from my grandmother's funeral. I can still smell the white lily and rose arrangements. I can hear the notes resonating off the harpist's hands. And I can still remember looking up at my mother, wondering why she was crying.

Hardly four years later, I would sit at the same gravesite to bury my grandfather after his lengthy battle with Parkinson's. Then, just months after his funeral, I would miss nearly half of my fifth-grade year to be with my aunt as ovarian cancer silently wove its way through her body before returning to the same cemetery again for the third time—all before my eleventh birthday.

Like many who feel called to healthcare, I wanted to help relieve the pain that I had to endure in my own life, and that I had seen others endure around me. Yet, like a recurring nightmare, these moments became ever present in my life. While I was sometimes able to relieve that pain under the right circumstances, too often my efforts were too little, too late. When I lie awake at night, I can still see the faces of the countless people I couldn't save from their inevitable fate. I can see the faces of their families, wondering why this had to happen to them.

However, it is those sleepless nights that have led me to uncover my ultimate vision in life. *I want to help people live longer, healthier, and more impactful lives.* It has taken time, reflection, and a long journey of self-education after my formal medical training to finally realize that this is absolutely possible, but only by working outside of the traditional healthcare industry. Which is why I'm writing this book.

The approach of traditional Western medicine is highly reactive. Doctors are essentially trained to wait until something goes wrong, and patients cross their fingers while relying upon highly specialized practitioners to treat their individual problems. That is, if they're caught in time—which they're often not. This is a convoluted, inefficient solution to an inherently simple problem. There *has* to be a better way.

It is becoming clearer that the array of seemingly niche diseases treated by subspecialized doctors all stem from the same underlying mechanisms—nearly all of which accelerate or cause premature cellular aging in the body. As we age, the organ systems in our bodies begin to falter and eventually break down altogether. While this results in the familiar wrinkles and gray hair, that's merely an external reflection of what is happening beneath.

When premature cellular aging is allowed to continue or even accelerate—which the standard American lifestyle all but ensures—we experience a host of chronic diseases that lead to rapid cognitive decline and physical frailty, which have a massive impact on our future, not just as individuals but as a society. Decreased productivity, poor sleep, increased stress, and the inability to show up for what matters is just the start. Diabetes, high blood pressure, heart disease, and obesity follow. As a result, we end up strapped to a runaway train barreling toward a ravine of heart attacks, strokes, dementia, and certain premature death.

Rather than waiting until something goes wrong and trying to fix it after the fact, the far more logical approach would be to use the abundance of knowledge we already have to slow or even stop cellular aging altogether, preventing many of these conditions from occurring in the first place. Unfortunately, our current medical system (at least in the United States) does not incentivize this type of behavior from doctors. There are no insurance reimbursement codes for truly preventative medicine, and the few that exist don't pay nearly what a procedure or "sick" visit does. Doctors are trained and paid to solve the problems in front of them—to keep their patients alive at all costs, not to educate them on how to prevent these problems twenty years before they take place. This practice is ineffective and only serves to perpetuate the cycle of unhealthy behavior, leading to an endless loop of further problems.

I'm here to tell you that *you have the power to stop that runaway train*. Your health outcomes are largely in your control, perhaps more than you might think. Heart attacks, strokes, cognitive decline, neurodegenerative diseases like Alzheimer's and Parkinson's...these are not the inevitable result of time, barring rare exceptions. They are the result of your lifestyle choices, environment, and circumstances throughout your life.

If you can slow the rate at which your body ages, you can prevent or significantly reduce the majority of chronic diseases that shorten not just your **lifespan** (how long you live), but your **healthspan** (how long you remain fit and functioning well). By implementing an intentional lifestyle focused on optimizing sleep, nutrition, mental wellness and physical movement, you can take control of your life, harness the full power of your brain and body, and avoid the fate of so many who succumb to these avoidable problems.

There's a growing mountain of evidence showing that many of these chronic diseases can be largely avoided through simple lifestyle changes. In addition to extending your lifespan, these intentional changes will also improve your performance, both mentally and physically, meaning you can accomplish more and feel better throughout your life, even well into your later years.

I've spent the recent years of my career trying to understand this evidence and how it can be used to change people's lives for the better. This book is the culmination of that knowledge.

HOW TO USE THIS BOOK

In the following chapters, I will arm you with a host of information you can use to increase your chance of living a longer and healthier life. Given my background as a clinical neurologist, I will be placing an emphasis on brain health in the hope that you may not only live longer but retain and even improve your cognitive function for as long as possible. As you'll soon discover, brain health and physical health are intimately intertwined, which is why so much of the information we'll cover relates to physical health in general. If things like resistance training, blood pressure, or nutrition don't seem relevant to the brain, these connections will soon be clear.

In Chapter 1, we'll clarify why you want to live longer in the first place. This is where many people fall short—they never connect their health to a deeper life mission, so they never make any lasting adjustments and the train keeps accelerating. There's now evidence that people with a clear purpose in life do, in fact, live longer.

By the end of that chapter, you should have a much clearer idea of what your purpose is and how that might impact decisions around your health. This idea of purpose will be a recurring theme throughout the book, which will serve as the motivation that will help you adhere to any and all of the lifestyle changes you choose to implement.

My approach is not to simply give you a list of recommendations, but to educate you on how your brain and body work and age, as well as why certain interventions are effective in slowing that rate of aging. That is why, after Chapter 1, the book is split into two parts: "Part 1: The Mechanisms" and "Part 2: The Interventions". Part 1 explains how many important age-related mechanisms work inside your body. We'll start with a primer on the brain, then move into four of the most common preventable causes of premature death before diving deep into the twelve hallmarks of aging.

In Part 2, we'll discuss the interventions that have been shown to lower your risk of developing many of the conditions discussed in Part 1. We'll start with the four big pillars of longevity (exercise, nutrition, sleep, and stress management) and cover some evidence-based principles for how to optimize these areas of your life. Next, we'll move on to the more peripheral (but still important) interventions like supplements, technology, and the future of medicine.

My goal with this book is to empower you to make more informed choices about your health, regardless of age or current health status. Whether you're in your thirties and looking to avoid chronic disease later in life or you're in your sixties and want to ensure you can make the most of your retirement, the information here applies to you. While it's true that the earlier you start implementing many of these interventions, the better your outcomes will likely be, *it's never too late to start*. Even small changes made later in life can have significant impacts on both your healthspan and lifespan. I have personally seen many patients undergo remarkable transformations in their later years that have undoubtedly added years to their lives.

I'd like to also clarify that most of the specific health challenges, statistics, and cultural factors I reference are largely drawn from my experience as a clinical neurologist practicing in the United States. Readers outside the US may find that some statistics differ in their countries, though the mechanisms, interventions, and the science remain broadly applicable, regardless of where you reside in the world.

As we dive into those mechanisms and interventions, you'll discover how many of these age-related conditions occur and why they are almost entirely preventable, including exactly *why* specific interventions can be so effective. I've done my best to simplify these concepts for those without medical backgrounds while also providing more specific details for those who are interested in going deeper. However, it should be noted that even the "in-depth" versions of these concepts are still wildly simplified—it would take multiple textbooks to explain many of these concepts, and if that's what you're looking for, you might as well just enroll in medical school.

In some places, I may offer you the option to skip ahead if you'd like to avoid the medical jargon. You're welcome to do that, although I'd suggest giving it an honest try before bailing out—you might just find it more interesting than you'd think. By understanding what's happening in your body at a cellular level, you'll also understand why certain interventions are beneficial and are therefore more likely to lead you to adopt healthy habits. Critically, you'll be well equipped to make better decisions around your health in the future as we learn more about the body and new interventions are discovered.

Even a general knowledge of these concepts will give you the ability to create your *own* longevity framework—one that works for you and your unique needs, preferences, and lifestyle. By understanding the foundations of a healthy lifestyle, you'll be able to decide what you want to implement and what you would rather do without—like a cold shower, perhaps.

This is my ultimate goal: for you to craft your own framework that works for you. I am by no means suggesting you implement everything I've discussed, and I won't be telling you exactly which foods to eat or what exercise routine to follow, for example. I'm merely presenting you with a framework of evidence-based information and interventions to consider. You're free to do with that what you will.

Some people may choose to implement everything in this book, which may serve them well. Others may only take just one tactic from this—which is great for them, too, because every little bit helps. Even if you dropped this book right now and simply walked away with a renewed motivation around developing a sustainable healthy lifestyle, I would chalk that up as a win.

The reality is that most people have a general sense of what they should be doing to live a healthier lifestyle. The problem for most people is a lack of confidence or urgency to change their lifestyle. I've watched this story play out time and time again in my own life and career. The vast majority of patients who end up in the hospital are there because, for one reason or another, they haven't prioritized their health over the course of their lives. And to be clear, this isn't their fault—our modern environment is set up to work against us from a health perspective. Busy schedules, constant stress, and the widespread availability of processed foods are just a few of many factors that make consistently healthy choices difficult.

This has been in the back of my mind throughout my entire career, but it's not something I could easily address. Understandably, most people don't want to hear that their loved one just died of something that was well within their control. For years, I grappled with this. It wasn't until one pivotal moment in my life that I decided enough was enough and chose to quit clinical medicine to pursue my vision and help more people. I feel compelled to share that moment with you, as it changed the course of my life forever.

MY BEST FRIEND

My lifelong best friend, Tanner, was one of the most influential people I've ever known. He was deeply introspective and keenly aware of his natural abilities—one of those people who seemed to just be naturally great at everything he did. He could get along with anyone, and he had an unearthly gift for making those around him feel comfortable. Tanner was one of these people you'd meet and somehow felt like you had known him your entire life.

Despite his natural abilities, Tanner struggled for years with his path in life. He was on a trajectory toward a lucrative career in the financial industry, yet deep down he felt something was missing. He couldn't ignore his call to join the ministry.

I distinctly remember a conversation we had in college, when he told me, "Ryan, I really don't want to do this, but I can't ignore God calling me."

In typical Tanner fashion, he found a way to do both. He believed he could minister to people from anywhere—even from the desk of a

Fortune 500 company—and so he did. To prepare, he studied abroad at universities across the globe, graduating *magna cum laude* with a degree in international and cultural studies, after which he pursued his theological education at Emory University's Candler School of Theology.

Tanner's greatest gift was the ability to make others feel seen and uniquely valued. Hours of conversation would pass until you realized he had masterfully guided you to share your deepest thoughts and concerns through his extraordinary ability to remain present and listen without judgment.

Unsurprisingly, after just a year of being appointed as a local pastor in his church, he was granted provisional eldership. He served for six years in this role before being ordained and appointed as an elder in the United Methodist Church on June 8, 2024, the crowning achievement of a ten-year journey.

Two days later, my phone rang. The vibrant green mountains outside my cabin window remain forever etched in my memory as I listened to our mutual friend Caleb struggle to find the words to tell me that Tanner had unexpectedly passed away in his home that afternoon.

In an instant, Tanner as we knew him ceased to exist.

As unbearable as the pain was to lose arguably the most steadfast and influential figure who had been present my entire life, Tanner's passing opened up another deep reflection. I asked myself questions like: Why am I really here? What is my purpose? Am I making a meaningful difference in the world?

Looking backward and connecting the dots of my life, I had an epiphany. I realized I have been allowed to suffer so that I can more fully understand the pain that others endure to know them better and be in a better position to help them.

In observing the arc of my life, through all the victories and tragedies, I finally realized that I am equipped and fully capable of helping people find more success in theirs. Through extensive work I have done on myself through years of therapy to overcome past trauma and limiting childhood beliefs, and in putting into practice much of the evidence-based lifestyle interventions we will discuss, I have become an entirely different person. Rather than hide behind a veil of insecurity, I am able to more deeply appreciate myself for all my strengths and my flaws. Rather than stifle my emotions, I am able to more fully express myself. And rather than remain guarded behind the armor of a white coat, I have become a better doctor, able to more fully see and heal my patients.

In a strange way, Tanner's passing was somehow his greatest and final gift.

In the wake of these deeply moving experiences, I have achieved ultimate clarity on my vision, my values, and my mission. Through the commitment I made to myself, I have written this book and started a company, Transcend Health, dedicated to improving the lives of others—which includes you. I am keeping true to my word, continuing to spread my message to help as many people as I am able. All this has become possible by putting science into practice, and I am here to tell you that this same power resides deep within you too—the power to realize your full potential.

Recently, I met another fellow neurologist, Anil, who, after hearing my story, told me of the time he met the Dalai Lama. While in his presence, a fellow bystander asked, "How can I help change the world? Everyone is so distracted, hurt, and selfish. What can I do to help them?"

His Holiness simply smiled and responded, "First, change yourself. Only then can the world change."

We are about to embark upon a journey through your brain, body, and the mechanisms that ultimately come together to form this beautiful symphony we call life. I am here to help guide you into the best version of yourself—physically, mentally, and emotionally—so that you too can go change the world.

Here's to your journey.

With love,
Ryan

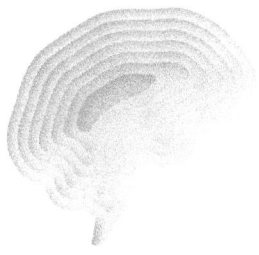

CHAPTER 1
FIND YOUR WHY

AS A DOCTOR, there are certain patients you simply never forget. Robert was one of those patients. I met Robert when he was 103 years old, during a dermatology rotation in my fourth year of medical school. I was just twenty-five and still in the early stages of my training, but I had already seen enough to realize there was something different about him and his wife, Laura.

Robert was the oldest patient I had seen up to that point, yet he and Laura strolled into the clinic on their own two feet with smiles on their faces. I am certain that every patient I had seen over the age of ninety up to that point required the assistance of a walker or wheelchair, was dealing with a multitude of significant health conditions, and would typically share some story about a spouse having recently passed away. Yet here were Robert and Laura, with nearly 200 years between them, practically skipping into the clinic like celebrities. (I later came to find out they *were* treated like celebrities because of how different they truly were from the average patient.)

I couldn't help myself. I had to know how they had achieved such an improbable feat. I felt something so profoundly different radiating from these two that transcended their already impressive health on paper, and I was dying to know what it was. So, with genuine curiosity, I asked both of them, "What's your secret?"

Robert responded playfully. "Well, we go dancing at least three times a week, and we're always the last couple there! I play golf just as often, and I even have friends on the PGA tour." I was already in awe, but what Robert said next would stay with me forever.

He leaned forward, looked me square in the eye, and told me something I would never forget. "You have to wake up every day with a *purpose*."

From that point on, I would make it a habit to ask all my older patients this same question. What's their secret? What had they done to make it this far in life, and in many cases, in such great shape? While I've received some interesting answers over the years, like "a shot of whiskey keeps the doctor away," or "too much fun with too many women causes real trouble," there's one consistent theme above all else: *maintaining a purpose.*

Before we dive into the "how" of living longer and feeling better, we need to spend a little time with the "why." Throughout this book, I'll walk you through some of the core science behind how your brain and body age, including what we actually know about preventing the physical and cognitive decline that so many people assume are inevitable (but isn't). We'll talk about what causes diseases like Alzheimer's, what's really happening when you step into a sauna, and yes, why everyone keeps talking about omega-3s. My goal here isn't to overwhelm you with biology, but to give you just enough understanding to make the rest of this book make sense—and to show you what's possible when you know how your body actually works.

While all that information is critical, I feel compelled to start this book with perhaps the most important piece of information I can offer. There's one concept that I believe is the cornerstone of nearly everything else when it comes to maximizing your longevity.

It is the one thing that affects all others—both physical and mental health, your cognitive function, even your own personal enjoyment and fulfillment.

IT IS THE IDEA OF *PURPOSE*

What I've discovered, both in my own life and through the lives of my patients, is that having a deep sense of purpose is perhaps the single greatest differentiating factor in separating those who make it into excellent health in their later years and those who don't. People who have a clear sense of purpose tend to wake up every day motivated to take intentional actions that are congruent with their goals. They see value in maintaining their health and optimizing their minds because doing so moves them closer to their desired outcomes. Their daily actions are thoughtfully planned and highly intentional because they are connected to an idea much bigger than themselves. Perhaps equally importantly, they tend to live life to the fullest and actually enjoy more of their time on earth, which markedly improves their quality of life—and, given what we know of how this affects the body, also very likely adds years to their life, as well.

This is not just anecdotal or conjecture on my part. There have been studies demonstrating that individuals with a deep sense of purpose have substantially improved odds at living longer. A 2019 study in *JAMA*, for example, looked at nearly 7,000 people with varying levels of self-reported purpose in their life. Over a four-year period, those who reported the lowest scores for life purpose were more than twice as likely to die from any cause. A 2022 study in the journal *Preventive Medicine* that examined over 13,000 people demonstrated a nearly 34 percent reduction in all-cause mortality in women and a 20 percent reduction in men when comparing the highest versus lowest levels of self-reported purpose.

This is not just a subjective idea that seems to move the needle. Having an elevated sense of purpose likely translates to lower levels of physical and mental stress, which leads to improved mental health, thereby lowering inflammation in the body, improving cardiovascular health, increasing resilience, improving levels of physical activity, and ultimately helping you retain cognitive and physical function for far longer.

All-cause mortality refers to the total number of deaths from any cause in a given population. When researchers say something has been shown to lower all-cause mortality, what they're really saying is that the evidence shows people who do that thing tend to live longer lives overall, regardless of what ultimately causes their death.

I believe having a clear purpose is the missing link in human longevity, and it is one of many cases where traditional Western medicine has failed us as a society. Unfortunately, most primary care doctors don't talk to their patients about this because our medical system offers no incentive for providers to do so. Really, our current "healthcare" model is more like a "sick care" model, through which doctors are paid to perform procedures and prescribe medications to people who are coming to them with a multitude of chronic illnesses.

Unlike many medical schools that focus exclusively on the **biomedical** model—emphasizing diagnosis and treatment of specific conditions—I was fortunate to train in a program where the curriculum is built around the **biopsychosocial** model. This approach views health through a more holistic lens, considering not just the biological factors, but also one's psychological needs and social determinants that affect their wellbeing, including an individual's sense of purpose.

Even though I received this formal training, once I started practicing I quickly realized how unrealistic this was to consistently implement because of the way our healthcare system is set up. This is one of a multitude of reasons that I chose to step away from clinical medicine to write this book and build my own healthcare business, Transcend Health. You can't talk to people about longevity without talking about *why* they want to live longer.

So, why *do* you want to live longer? What is your purpose in life? This will be our first order of business together, and I'd like you to keep it in mind as you read on. Toward the end of this chapter, we're going to come back to it. Your goal should be to have further clarity on your purpose (ideally in a written statement) by the end of this chapter, because everything we'll cover from here on out will relate back to it.

In the meantime, however, I'd like to provide some context for why you're reading this, what "longevity" really means, and what we're going to be doing together.

WHY LIVE LONGER?

The fact that you've picked up this book is no surprise. Throughout the course of written history, we humans have been fascinated by the idea of prolonging life. This has most commonly taken the form of the proverbial "Fountain of Youth," waiting to be discovered in some far-off land.

One of the earliest known mentions of this concept comes from the Greek historian Herodotus, in the fifth century BCE. Herodotus told the story of the Macrobians, an ancient people who lived in the horn of Africa—an area as distant to the Ancient Greeks as the moon might be to us. The Macrobians, Herodotus claimed, were renowned for their physical beauty, towering stature, and above all, their astonishing longevity. They were said to live to 120 years old, allegedly by drinking from a sacred, life-giving river. Its waters were described as "sweet and light," unlike the brackish waters of other lands. Perhaps their impressive lifespans were simply a result of drinking clean water at a time when sanitary conditions were abysmal, although I think it's more likely Herodotus was telling a tall tale.

This same theme, however, is found across many cultures throughout history. Perhaps my favorite example is that of Juan Ponce de León, the Spanish explorer commissioned by King Ferdinand in 1512 to settle the island of Bimini, which was rumored to be a land of riches and wonder. He ultimately landed near St. Augustine, Florida, and legend has it that he discovered the Fountain of Youth there. In typical Florida fashion, there's now a tourist attraction where visitors can drink from the supposed fountain. As a native Floridian, I've done this, and I can't say I recommend it. The water smells like sulfur and I have yet to notice any benefits. Although, maybe this is the *real* reason retirees flock to Florida in droves. Here I was thinking it was the weather....

The fact that these legends have endured to this day demonstrates that longevity is central to the human condition—and clearly this fascination hasn't slowed down. Over the last several hundred years, and especially in the past several decades, there's been an explosion of technological and scientific advances in medicine, particularly within the field of longevity.

Besides the obvious monumental advances in medical science like the (accidental) discovery of penicillin by Alexander Fleming and the development of vaccines, as a society we've collectively invested billions of dollars into research around increasing human longevity. The "longevity industry"—which encompasses disciplines like biotechnology, regenerative medicine, preventive healthcare, and a host of wellness innovations—is projected to grow to $120 billion by 2032. I suppose you and I are now part of that!

Clearly, most of us have some innate desire to live a longer life, preserve our youth, and in some cases even achieve immortality. But *why?* Is this a unique feature of being human? Or perhaps something hard-wired into our DNA?

If we adopt an evolutionary perspective, living longer increases the probability that you can bear offspring and propagate your genes, which is directly in line with Darwin's theory of natural selection, favoring survival of the fittest. The fact that you exist is a testament to this, as some of the most successful genes to ever exist reside within you right now. You have already defied incredible odds just by being alive at a moment in history when 99 percent of all species to ever exist on our planet are now extinct. So, yes, it is fair to say that a desire for longevity *is* hard-wired into your DNA.

Beyond that, living longer and in good health offers countless intrinsic benefits to society:

- Healthier populations create more productive workforces, reduce healthcare costs, and drive innovation
- When people maintain better health for longer, they build stronger relationships and communities, creating support networks that benefit everyone
- The longer we live, the more experience and information we can pass on to younger generations

The healthier we are as individuals, the healthier and more successful we become as a collective society.

OUR HEALTH PARADOX

If an alien were to land on earth and read up to this point, they'd be right in thinking that the human population must be living longer, healthier lives than ever before. *Finally,* after thousands of years of a near-zero increase in the average human lifespan, we now have the tools to affect meaningful change on this front. We have the knowledge, medicines, and interventions necessary to live far longer, healthier lives than even our grandparents! So we *must* be healthier than ever before, right?

While it's true that life expectancy has increased by approximately two and a half years per decade since the 1840s, equivalent to an extra three months for every year we are alive, the sad reality is that the overall health of our population is in frightening decline, especially in the United States. For starters, 93 percent of Americans are considered metabolically unhealthy, meaning that the overwhelming majority of us are not within optimal ranges for body weight, cholesterol, blood pressure, or fat and sugar levels in our bloodstream. This is a serious problem due to the chronic diseases that directly result from these underlying problems, which unsurprisingly affect two thirds of Americans. 74 percent of us are overweight or obese, which leads to more chronic health conditions. 92 percent of us have at least one micronutrient deficiency—and micronutrients are critical for our basic cellular functions. And the kicker is, *nearly all these conditions are preventable!*

Heart disease, for example, is the leading cause of death in the US and is almost entirely preventable just by living an intentionally healthy lifestyle. This appears evident from the mountain of data we've collected on the subject, but you can also discern this by looking at nature. Believe it or not, heart disease is an almost exclusively *human* disease. By and large, wild animals do not suffer from narrowed arteries, high blood pressure, or heart attacks.

Why might this be the case? It's almost certainly due to their lifestyle. In contrast to humans, animals in the wild move constantly, eat a natural and unprocessed diet, don't smoke, avoid heavy levels of pollution (although humans have greatly threatened this), and don't experience chronic stress. As you'll see in Chapter 3, consistent exercise alone is enough to drastically lower your risk of heart disease, and yet in the United States alone, someone still dies of a heart attack about every thirty seconds.

You might think I wouldn't see the effects of these conditions as a neurologist, but I most certainly do. Most of my career has been spent in hospitals across the country, caring for people suffering from neurologic emergencies such as acute strokes and the debilitating symptoms of neurodegenerative diseases. Like heart disease, these are largely preventable problems—yet every three minutes someone dies of a stroke in the US. Every day I work at the hospital, the overhead code pages signal the same morbid words: "code stroke" and "code blue," indicating a life-threatening stroke or heart attack, respectively. It's practically nonstop. It saddens me and quite frankly, I'm tired of it.

So, let me be clear:

THE LENGTH AND QUALITY OF YOUR LIFE ARE LARGELY WITHIN YOUR CONTROL

Heart attacks, strokes, dementia, and many of the life-altering conditions we fear are often seen or learned as being entirely out of our control. Some of the common narratives I encounter are: "It's just luck"; "It's genetics"; "My father has dementia so that's what will happen to me."

This is largely false. The reality is that somewhere between 70–90 percent of all health outcomes are lifestyle-based, meaning genetics are part of the equation but play a much smaller role than you think—not to mention, with genome editing technologies like CRISPR in the works, your genes will likely play even *less* of a role in the future.

Other than avoiding an unexpected accident or inheriting a rare genetic condition, luck has little to do with it. Chronic diseases don't just randomly show up in your body one day; they're almost always the cumulative result of your environment, your circumstances, and the actions you've taken throughout your life—many of which can have negative consequences that go unnoticed until they manifest themselves in an extreme way, like a heart attack or stroke. Even diagnoses that you may have previously thought were out of your control, such as developing Alzheimer's or Parkinson's later in life, can be almost entirely prevented just by making the right choices on a daily basis.

So, if we have more tools at our disposal to improve our health than ever before...and we know exactly what's killing us...and these things can be prevented...*why on earth are so many people dying prematurely and suffering from a multitude of chronic diseases?*

THE CARDS ARE STACKED AGAINST US

In today's world, most people are generally aware of what they need to do to live a long life. In fact, I'll go ahead and give you the secret to longevity right now: *eat well, exercise regularly, lower your stress, and get good sleep.* But you already knew that, didn't you?

So, the question becomes: Why doesn't everyone just do those things? Why, given all the knowledge and tools we finally have at our disposal, do we still live largely unhealthy lifestyles? Why are hospitals inundated with people suffering from the debilitating effects of chronic diseases that are entirely preventable?

Throughout my career, I have found that information alone is not the deciding factor in whether someone lives a healthy lifestyle or not (and yes, I realize the irony of that statement as I write a book filled to the brim with information). The hardest part for most people is actually following through with the steps required to live longer. Committing to regular exercise, eating well, keeping stress low, and sleeping well on a consistent basis over the course of decades is *hard,* make no mistake about it. And it has become even harder in modern society, where the game seems like it is practically rigged against you.

The scary reality is that corporations and entire industries have discovered how to hijack your brain. Social media "likes," never-ending video feeds, processed foods fortified with sugar, one-click shopping with same-day delivery, pornography, the twenty-four-hour news cycle, addictive substances...these things are by no means good for your intrinsic health, but like a moth to a flame, you gravitate toward them because they activate the primitive pleasure and fear circuits in your brain. Corporations know this and quite literally have teams of people who design products engineered to take advantage of these circuits. I would like to believe this wasn't initially done with malevolent intent, but the results are unfortunately the same.

A **circuit** or **neural circuit** is a network of interconnected neurons within the brain that work together to process information and guide behavior. In other words, a group of brain cells operating in tandem to perform a specific function, like moving or talking.

I tell you this not to frighten or demoralize you, but to make one thing abundantly clear: *none of this is your fault.* It is not your fault that you just wasted twenty minutes scrolling on social media without realizing it. It is not your fault that you finished that bag of chips when you had every intention of pacing yourself. It is not your fault that you'd rather watch TV than go to the gym. It doesn't mean you lack willpower or self-control, and it certainly doesn't mean you're a bad person. You do these things because they're intentionally designed to take advantage of the way your brain functions.

To fully understand how this works, let's take a brief detour to the brain. Deep within your brain exists a primitive set of structures called the limbic system. This complex arrangement is found in nearly all animals, and within it exists a reward system that is designed to encourage you to do more of the things that benefit you and less of the things that don't. This system was originally designed to ensure your ancestors' survival. It provided the motivation to continue working hard in anticipation of completing a task such as finding food and a little extra boost once that task was complete.

This inherited reward system functions largely through the chemical messenger, **dopamine.** Dopamine is the principal neurotransmitter responsible for making you feel good, and rather than dopamine only being released when "good" things happen, your brain actually releases it largely in anticipation of a reward.

Think about something you really wanted in the past—maybe a new toy as a child or an upcoming vacation as an adult—and how excited you were right up until the moment you received it or stepped on the plane. Typically, it's a bit anticlimactic once you achieve the desired object, which reflects the relative levels of dopamine involved on either side of the equation. This system makes logical sense, or at least it did at one point in our evolution, as it helped our ancestors become conditioned to seek more of something that might help ensure their survival, like food, procreation, and shelter.

The modern problem with this system is that dopamine-producing neurons don't just fire when you receive a reward. They also respond to a condition termed a **reward prediction error.** This means that they fire more strongly when you receive a reward that is better than expected, and less strongly when you receive a reward that is worse than expected, which is largely how you learn to adjust your behavior based on your experiences. In essence, your brain becomes conditioned to subconsciously prioritize activities that reward you with the highest amount of dopamine for the least amount of effort.

Nowadays, all you have to do is pull your smartphone out of your pocket as you scroll through an endless feed of wildly engaging videos while sitting in the drive-thru lane at your favorite fast food establishment, ready to binge on an array of ultra savory and sweet extra-sized meal combos—all of which flood your brain with excess dopamine, ultimately creating a subconscious pattern of addiction. As a result, you're unknowingly reinforcing predictable behaviors that keep you returning to and paying for these services, resulting in massive profits for companies and a compensatory decline in your overall health. It is *in your nature* to fall into these habits because of the disproportionate reward signal they provide. As far as your brain is concerned, you're doing the right thing.

And therein lies the problem. The reward system that once helped your ancestors survive—and, ironically, ensured your existence in the first place—is now perhaps your greatest threat. Building the habits to ensure you perform the activities which are *actually* beneficial—like eating a whole food, unprocessed diet and exercising, to start—do not initially provide nearly the same reward signal as what you may be accustomed to, like watching videos of cats chasing laser beams or my niece's TikTok with over seven million views (which is a true story, and I'm very proud of her). But the key word is "initially"...

REBALANCING THE EQUATION

The good news is that you can essentially rebalance your reward system by training yourself to anticipate the good that will come from beneficial activities, which can in turn provide their own source of reward and pleasure for your brain. Not to mention, once you experience the near immediate improvement in your mood, physical health, and overall performance, this will create even greater anticipation of having more of the "right" stuff in your life.

So, what's the best way to get started?

We can start by eliminating a few methods that *don't* work. Making drastic health changes overnight or setting overly ambitious goals have clearly been shown *not* to work. (There's a reason why the second day of January is called "Quitter's Day.") Setting vague goals like "getting healthy" or "losing my belly fat" have also been shown to be ineffective over the long term. Relying solely on willpower is not an effective tactic either, and a surefire way to feel guilty about your progress as motivation ebbs and flows.

What *does* work, however, is making incremental changes and sticking with them, allowing you to reap the benefits that compound over time. While a broad range exists, studies have shown that it takes sixty-six days, on average, to fully adopt a new habit, although it doesn't have to take nearly this long. Therefore, the best way to incorporate healthy habits is to start small, make it easy for yourself, and focus on one thing at a time.

Focusing on activities you enjoy will also substantially increase the chance that you keep doing them, which is really all that matters. Perhaps most importantly, every little bit counts and it's *never* too late to start. Don't beat yourself up if you're not perfect. Any amount of progress is better than no progress, and every decision you make is an investment in your future health.

It should be said that this book and the interventions in it are not going to change your life overnight (well, getting better sleep might, but that's about it). In terms of your brain and body, there are no "quick fixes" or "life hacks." There are only intentional habits you can choose to implement that serve your ultimate purpose and end goal, or not. Therefore, my goal is to help you embrace a new, better way of living by making consistent, sustainable, incremental changes and transforming them into habits. As Aristotle allegedly once said, "We are what we repeatedly do. Excellence, therefore, is not an act but a habit." What he may not have known is the massive impact our habits have on the quality and duration of our lives.

Throughout our time together, my focus will be on making things as easy as possible and taking them one step at a time. With a deeper knowledge of how you operate, you'll understand *why* certain interventions are beneficial and will therefore be more likely to implement and adhere to them. You'll learn how to design your environment and lifestyle to reshape your behavior, allowing you to work with your brain's natural tendencies rather than against them. And you'll ultimately be able to use neuroscience to your advantage, stacking the cards in *your* favor, not against you as you have unknowingly been accustomed to.

All this can lead to a longer, healthier life in which you're able to do more of the things you love. This is perhaps the best gift you could ever give yourself. Those far-off dreams you've had since you were a child are achievable. You can travel the world in your later years in excellent health. You can not only *watch* your grandchildren grow up but *be an active part of their lives.*

Prioritizing your health is also perhaps the most selfless thing you could do, because showing up for the world in your best and fullest capacity—the way you were meant to—allows you to make an even greater impact on others. These things are all within your control, and that realization is the first step in the process.

The main vessel for this change, however, begins with your purpose. Why do you want to live longer? Why do you want to prioritize your health? What is your end goal? Understanding your purpose provides the underlying motivation that allows you to sustain those incremental changes over time. Without a compelling reason for you to stay the course, your brain is likely to fall into the same predictable traps.

PURPOSE AND LEGACY

At the beginning of this chapter, I asked you to consider your purpose in life. It's time to come back to that. Achieving clarity about your purpose provides the single greatest chance for you to live longer and increase your impact on the world.

When you think about it, living longer without a sense of purpose is kind of meaningless. What benefit do a handful more months or years serve you if you don't have something to live for? I witnessed the profound impact this can have during the later years of my paternal grandfather's life. For ninety-four years, Papa had a clear sense of purpose in his life: he was a fighter pilot, professional race car driver, orthopedic surgeon, husband, and father of five. He was connected to goals much bigger than himself, with targets to aim for (sometimes literally, as a fighter pilot) and countless reasons to exist long into his future.

When my grandmother passed away from leukemia, however, he only stuck around for another twenty-eight days. When she left, so did his sense of purpose. He had nothing left to live for. You've surely heard similar stories about elderly couples passing away shockingly close to each other. It's something I've seen countless times with my patients, but losing two dearly beloved family members in close succession painfully drove this lesson home and is a clear indicator that having a purpose matters.

But this is not something that only affects us later in life. People with a clear sense of purpose are typically more active throughout their lives, which has also been consistently reproduced in studies. They don't sit on the couch all day because they have things to do and places to be. As a result, they're also typically more socially active, which has a number of benefits for brain health and physical health (which in many ways are one and the same, given the mechanisms that underlie each, as we will discover).

Regularly exploring new environments—in location and conversation—allows people to actively engage and continuously challenge their minds, which helps them retain their cognitive function for longer, and ultimately contributes to maintaining their healthspan. This deep-seated, intrinsic motivation that comes from having a strong sense of purpose also translates into prioritizing positive habits like exercise and avoiding negative habits like a sedentary lifestyle or consuming a poor diet. This is largely because these individuals understand that optimizing their bodies allows them to continue performing to the best of their abilities and accomplish more of what they set out to do.

Simply put, the more mentally and physically active you remain throughout your life, the longer you'll likely live, and with much higher levels of retained cognitive and physical function along the way. Therefore, perhaps the single greatest thing you can do for yourself and your long-term health is to take the time to find your purpose in life, as it will naturally lead you to better choices.

Now, clarifying a singular purpose for your entire life might sound like a daunting task—and it can be—but I've found it to be much easier than you might think. In my experience, when I ask people about their purpose, even though the answers are all different, they naturally emerge. While you may have never sat down and thought about it previously, you instinctively have a deep sense of what you want out of life. All you have to do is ask yourself the question.

One of the best ways I have found to help clarify your purpose is to start by thinking about your legacy. Legacy is typically thought of as something that happens to people after they're gone, but I'd argue that's not exactly the case. Your legacy is typically a summation of your impact on the world. Well...aren't you creating that impact right now?

Your legacy isn't something that magically appears after you die; it is something you are actively working on throughout your life. Your legacy is alive and well in this very moment, and your purpose is inherently tied to that legacy. What you choose to do every day in this life directly affects the legacy you continuously create while you're here and will ultimately leave when you're gone.

I'd like to go a little deeper with this, because I believe this might be the one concept that will flip the switch in your brain, creating the proverbial light-bulb moment with which we're all familiar. (And while there are no actual light bulbs in your brain, it might amaze you to know that your brain generates enough energy to power one! More to come on that in Chapter 2.)

Merriam-Webster defines legacy as "a gift by will, especially of money or other personal property." The second definition is "something transmitted by or received from an ancestor or predecessor or from the past." For our purposes, neither of these definitions will do, because legacy is about far more than personal property or the transmission of "things" between generations.

To me, legacy is many things. It's how you show up every day. It's who you become. It's not just some "thing" that materializes in your place after you're gone. Sure, your legacy is how people will remember you once you move on from this life, but that legacy is created by the actions, character, principles, and love that you take, develop, and give while you are alive.

The real light-bulb moment for me was the realization that these are the things you do *every single day*. It's the kind of spouse you are. The kind of parent you become. It's your friendships and your leadership at work. It's the impact you create. It's your philanthropy, which could be something as simple yet valuable as giving your time to others. The beauty is that your legacy changes as you change. Your abilities, interests, and environment shape how you respond to life and create new and different opportunities to optimize your legacy.

When we remove all the superficial layers and examine what really matters in this life, the most important things are not related to money, titles, or achievements. By far, among the most important and precious gifts we hold are the people closest to us, the impact we make on others, and the memories we leave them with. This is central to most people's legacy and therefore their purpose.

So, with that in mind, I encourage you to ask yourself:

- What impact do you want to make on the people around you?
- How do you want to serve and love others, even if they're complete strangers?
- What kind of world do you want to leave for your children or your grandchildren?
- What if you knew you could change the course of someone's life for the better with even a small gesture?

Changing the course of one person's life can create a ripple effect far beyond what you may ever fully see. The impact you make doesn't always manifest in obvious ways. It can happen through a moment of presence, a simple gesture, or a conversation that reaches someone at exactly the right time. Many times, we don't even realize the difference we've made until much later—if ever. But these small, human moments can reshape someone's trajectory in lasting, meaningful ways.

That's the heart of legacy: not something that happens after you're gone, but something you are actively creating now—in the way you show up, the choices you make, and the care you offer. When we talk about purpose, we're also talking about finding alignment with those deeper desires—to love, to serve, to build, to experience. And when you link your daily actions to those desires, even the smallest habits begin to carry deeper meaning. Because when you live from that place of intention, not only are you investing in your health and future—you're also building a life that reflects who you truly are and the impact you want to leave behind.

YOUR WHY

To make these concepts of purpose and legacy as practical as possible, I like to distill everything down into one simple why statement. This statement is your answer to the big question: Why do you want to live a longer, healthier life?

When you have clarity on the answer to this question—and when it is ever-present in your mind—the right choices become obvious. You naturally want to build sound habits to optimize your effectiveness and your ability to create meaningful impact. The right habits go from being things you *have to do* to things you *want to do* because you can easily connect them to the end result you've envisioned.

So, with that in mind, I'd like to present you with a choice right now. You have a choice to write down your why and use it to begin your journey toward a longer, healthier, and more impactful life. To make this as easy as possible, I've included an exercise on the following page (or available for download at TranscendHealthGroup.com/Resources) to help you get started. This, as you'll see, will be a common theme throughout the book. The easier you can make things for yourself, the more likely you are to do them. And along that same theme, the more ways your brain can interact with new information, the more likely you are to build robust connections to access and use it!

Every choice you make today is a vote for the world you want to live in tomorrow, and that choice starts right now.

FINDING YOUR WHY

Studies show that writing down your goals significantly increases the likelihood of achieving them. Take time to thoughtfully answer these questions, being specific where you can. Once complete, keep your why statement somewhere visible as a daily reminder.

PART 1: IMPACT AND ACHIEVEMENT

Impact Questions:

1. Who are the key people in your life who you want to impact? Think about family, friends, and mentors.

   _____
   _____
   _____

2. For the people listed above:
   - How do you want them to remember you?
   - What kind of impact do you want to have on their lives?
   - What experiences do you want to share with them?

3. Beyond your immediate circle, what communities or causes matter most to you?

_____
_____
_____

Achievement Questions:

1. What are your biggest dreams or goals? Be as specific as possible. Think about places you want to go, things you want to create, milestones you want to reach.

_____
_____
_____

2. What activities or work makes you feel most alive and fulfilled?

_____
_____
_____

3. Looking ahead to your later years, what do you want to be able to do? Think about both day-to-day activities and bigger achievements.

_____
_____
_____

PART 2: CREATING YOUR WHY STATEMENT

Using your answers above, write one to two sentences that capture:
- The people and communities you want to impact
- The key achievements you want to accomplish
- Why maintaining your health and longevity is essential to these goals

Your statement should feel personal and meaningful. When you read it, you should feel motivated to make choices that support a longer, healthier life.

Here are some examples of why statements from patients and other people I've worked with. As you'll see, they are very different from one another. That's the point! This brief sample is just for the purpose of getting you started. Your own why can be as extensive as you want it to be.

- *I want to watch my grandchildren grow up.*
- *I want to walk my daughter down the aisle.*
- *I want to help people achieve personal or financial freedom.*
- *I want to summit mountains on every continent.*
- *I want to build a business that makes the world a better place.*
- *I want to build a garden that will outlive me and nourish my family for generations.*
- *I want to remain independent and self-sufficient until the day I die.*
- *I want to visit over one hundred countries in my lifetime.*

KEY TAKEAWAYS

1. **Your why is your most powerful longevity tool.** Finding your deeper purpose and clarifying *why* you want to live longer creates intrinsic motivation that makes healthy choices sustainable. Your why is a combination of your purpose and legacy. Write it down and keep it at the forefront of your mind.

2. **You have significant control over your longevity.** Between 70–90 percent of your health outcomes are determined by lifestyle choices, not genetics or luck. Understanding that most chronic diseases are preventable through consistent habits empowers you to take ownership of your future health.

3. **Start with small, sustainable changes.** Rather than attempting dramatic overnight transformations, focus on incorporating manageable, incremental habits that align with your why. Create an environment that makes healthy choices easy, and develop one habit at a time until it becomes automatic before adding more. Every little bit helps.

PART 1

THE MECHANISMS

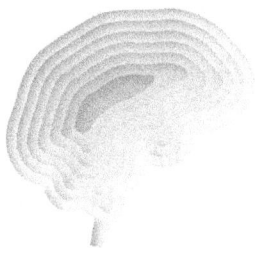

CHAPTER 2
THE BRAIN

THE ROCKS SKITTER away beneath John's feet as he skids to a stop at the cliff's edge. He watches as they tumble down over the cliff face, then, peering over, sees them splash into the water hundreds of feet below. His lungs burn and his mind races. Glancing back, his eyes widen with fear as the pack of wildebeest thunder toward him, a cloud of dust in their wake, the sound of their hooves nearly deafening.

The sun beats down. His lips and mouth are dry as he considers his options. With nowhere left to run, he knows he must either stand his ground or risk plunging into the depths below. He envisions each outcome—both painful, both potentially deadly. How deep is the water? Can he survive from this height? Will the wildebeest trample him? Or will they stop before the cliff's edge? With only seconds to come to a decision, he closes his eyes, tenses his entire body, and braces for impact.

And then: silence.

A moment of disorientation gives way to new sensations: cool air flowing gently across his face; the soft chirping of a wren in the distance; the faint smell of pancakes. As he turns over, John notices the familiar feeling of soft down and cotton brushing against his skin. A thin ray of morning light streams through the window, illuminating the familiar shapes of the nightstand, lamp, and writing desk that inhabit his bedroom.

As he checks his phone, John finally comes to the conscious realization that he is not, in fact, fighting for his life on the plains of Africa. He is safe, comfortably lying in his bed while his wife prepares breakfast downstairs. He's had another intense dream—so vivid, so *real*, that a part of him still feels as if he's in danger, even though the rational voice in his brain reassures him he isn't. With a heavy sigh, he rubs his eyes, pulls off the covers, and steps onto the floor. Another day begins.

This is just one example of the infinite and remarkably powerful experiences your brain can create. John just lived through an intense, lifelike simulation while his body was asleep. So lifelike, in fact, that his brainwave activity during that dream probably looked remarkably similar to what it would have if he were actually in that situation in real life. After he awoke, it even took a moment for him to realize that it was just a dream, which I'm sure you can relate to.

What's more, that cliff and those wildebeest existed only in the realm of your imagination as you read about them, yet you just visualized the entire scene complete with sensory details and emotional weight. You could feel the terror, sense the warmth of the sun, hear the thundering hooves, and feel the cool morning air in John's bedroom. You could visualize John's appearance, even though he is an entirely fictional character. And you were able to do all of this just by viewing a series of symbols on a page as your brain interpreted them in real time.

Your brain was able to accomplish this by utilizing the associations and references of your prior memories and experiences to create a simulation in your mind. This required little to no effort on your part—it just happened. And your brain accomplishes tasks like this thousands of times every single day. How incredible is that?

WELCOME TO THE INCREDIBLE BRAIN

In this chapter, we'll explore the human brain—the remarkable command center of your body that is currently decoding and processing the information on this page while simultaneously orchestrating an innumerable host of other complex functions to keep your body running. And while brain health is often thought to be separate from physical health, you'll soon learn how that couldn't be further from the truth.

The fact of the matter is that in many ways brain health *is* physical health, and vice versa. Nearly all the mechanisms and interventions we'll cover that relate to your physical health have an effect on your brain as well, because they are inherently intertwined. Not to mention, even if your body were in perfect health, without your brain you wouldn't think much of it anyway....

While I'm typically not one for absolutes, I feel comfortable saying that your brain is unequivocally the most important organ in your body. It's intimately involved in everything you do, it cannot be replaced, and it must be taken care of. Keeping your brain healthy by avoiding the many diseases known to affect it is one of the best ways to maximize the length of time you are able stay in top shape. Whatever your why is, I guarantee you'll want to retain your cognitive function for as long as possible so you can keep doing what matters! Therefore, it only makes sense to start your longevity journey with a basic understanding of your brain.

In this chapter we'll start with a broad overview of how your brain functions, then look at three critical systems within the brain that are essential for your longevity:

1. Learning and Memory
2. Motor Control
3. Emotional Regulation

While there are countless systems within your brain that we could discuss, a basic understanding of these three mechanisms will give you the best bang for your buck with respect to longevity. These three functions pose the largest detriment to your health if lost or damaged, and perhaps the greatest impact when optimized. Better yet, each of these systems can be maintained and even enhanced through simple lifestyle changes.

I'm going to give you my best oversimplified (but still kind of complex) explanation of how these parts of your brain work, because once you begin to understand how things work on a more micro level, you'll start to appreciate why certain interventions we discuss in the later chapters are so critically important.

To better illustrate this, it's time for a pop quiz! I've dropped a few questions below which I'll bring up again at the end of the chapter. After reading through, you should be able to easily answer these questions in your own words—and not coincidentally, you'll even understand how your brain is able to recall that information!

1. How does sleep affect memory retention?
2. How can blood pressure impact various systems in your brain?
3. How could a problem in the "motor control" system in your brain also affect memory retention?
4. Why is social activity beneficial for your brain?
5. Why might racquetball players live longer than others?
6. How can positive thinking impact your longevity?

THE POWER OF THE HUMAN BRAIN

I will never forget the first time I held a human brain. I was a sophomore in my undergraduate studies and fortunate enough to enroll in a neuroscience course taught by a professor at the medical school. I was one of just eight students in the entire class and Dr. Nolan poured into us that semester. The more he taught us about the brain, the more fascinated I became.

At the time it seemed almost impossible to comprehend just how complex our brains are—and the truth is, we *still* don't fully know how the brain works. While we've developed a deep understanding of how our brains function over the past two hundred years or so thanks to pioneers like Ramón y Cajal, Golgi, Charcot, and the like, we're still in the process of discovering how it all works, which is rapidly advancing thanks to continued improvements in technology.

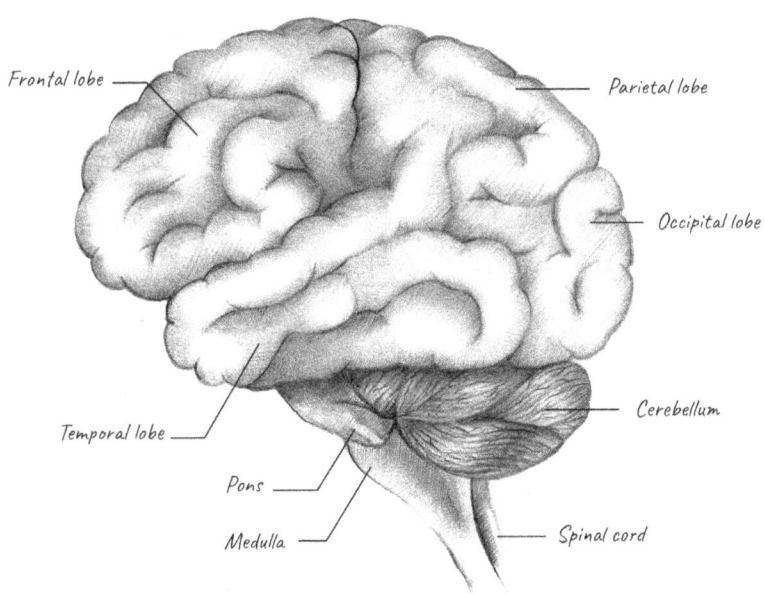

DIAGRAM 1: *The Brain*

For starters, your brain is an organ (not a muscle, despite what you might have heard) that receives 20 percent of your body's total energy supply despite accounting for only 2 percent of your entire body weight. Your kidney is the only other organ that even comes close.

I like to describe the brain as a complex collection of neurons, because that's quite literally what it is. A **neuron** is a specialized cell in your nervous system that processes and transmits information through electrical signals. There are around 86 billion neurons in your brain, all organized into unique patterns, with the majority of them residing in the gray matter on the outside of your brain, also known as the **cortex**. The rest are nestled deep within your brain into groups of cells called **nuclei**.

Almost everything in between is made of:

1. Wires or **axons** that connect all your neurons, also known as "white matter"
2. Another 50 billion **glial** or "support" cells that help maintain the environment of your neurons (think glial for glue)
3. The tiny blood vessels (arteries and veins) that supply your brain cells with blood
4. An intricate system of interconnected fluid-filled chambers designed to help filter out the waste products your brain accumulates throughout the day

Therefore, the total number of "brain cells" (neurons and glial cells) in your body is somewhere between 136 and 150 billion. Yes, that's billion with a "b".

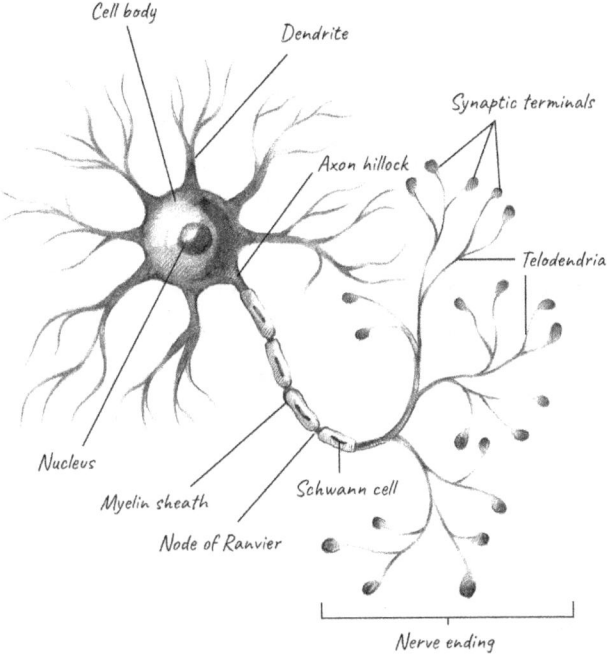

DIAGRAM 2: *Neuron + Glial Cell*

If you think that sounds like a lot, your neurons are connected to each other through what are known as **synapses**, and there are thought to be somewhere between 100 trillion and one quadrillion of these connections in your brain. (That's a one with seventeen zeros behind it if you, like me, have a hard time visualizing such a comically large number.) These synapses are what allow your neurons to communicate with each other, conveying information in the form of electrical impulses. Critically, these connections can be changed through a process called **neuroplasticity**, which is your brain's ability to change its structure and function in response to new experiences, injuries, or environmental cues.

Each individual neuron can have hundreds or even thousands of **dendritic spines**, which look like little arms that grow, recede, connect to, and communicate with thousands of other adjacent neurons. This is an important process to understand, because this is exactly what happens when you learn something new, and your brain modifies your behavior as a result. In fact, this is happening in your brain right now—those dendritic spines are connecting to and communicating with thousands of other neurons to create a unique neural pattern that will form your memory of this information. Wild, I know.

It's also worth noting that the electrical pulses we're referring to are really just small chemical reactions that are happening constantly across your entire brain. Each individual neuron is estimated to undergo 100,000 chemical reactions per second, which means that there are over 500 quadrillion chemical reactions blazing across your neurons every single minute—and that doesn't even include what's happening in the glial cells! I hope you're starting to see why neuroscience is so fascinating, and we haven't even scratched the surface.

For context, those chemical reactions collectively generate about twenty watts of power (one joule per second), which is enough to light up multiple LED bulbs, charge your smartphone, run your smartwatch, or even power your TV in sleep mode. From that electrochemical symphony emerges the beautiful experience we call human consciousness, which still eludes the ability of modern science to fully explain—although, at the time of writing, the advent of artificial intelligence and quantum computing may get us there sooner than we think.

THE BRAIN IS A PROCESSOR

All these reactions and connections allow your brain to process and decode a constant array of incoming information at an alarmingly fast rate. In other words, the human brain is nature's most sophisticated supercomputer.

It's important to note that your brain is more of a central processor than a receptor. Your body collects information in the billions of peripheral nerve cells that live outside your brain (in your skin and throughout your body) which then send that information to the brain for processing.

One way to conceptualize this is the simple fact that your brain does not actually feel pain, but your peripheral nerve cells that live in your skin and various organs do. For example, when you stub your toe, specialized nerve endings in your foot activate and transmit a signal through your foot, up your leg, through your spinal cord, and into your brain, where it is then decoded and processed. Only after that entire sequence of events has transpired do you experience the perception of pain, which can take between 200 to 400 milliseconds.

This is why patients are often intentionally left awake during brain surgery, so that when a neurosurgeon stimulates a particular area of the brain the patient is able to communicate where they perceive the sensation, such as their left arm tingling, or the urge to move their right thumb, which ultimately helps the surgeon minimize injury to important adjacent regions of the brain by knowing to avoid them.

By many estimates, your brain receives up to 11 million bits of information per second from your various sensory systems—visual, auditory, olfactory (smell), gustatory (taste), and tactile (touch). For comparison, this is roughly equivalent to the speed of a basic 100mbps home internet plan, which is more than enough bandwidth to stream multiple 4K movies on various devices simultaneously. (Whoa!)

Technically, there are eight total sensory systems. In addition to the five most of us know, you are also equipped with:
- **The vestibular system,** which allows you to sense balance
- **The proprioceptive system,** which allows you to sense movement from your muscles and joints and know where you are in space
- **The interoceptive system,** which allows you to sense internal stimuli such as pain, temperature, and stretch (this is how you feel full after a huge meal, for example)

Another interesting consideration is that even though your brain is receiving those 11 million bits per second, your conscious mind can only process about 50 bits per second, several orders of magnitude less.

Why might that be? For one, to conserve energy; your brain constantly filters this information and ignores anything that isn't worth sacrificing your attention. For example, you probably weren't aware of the precise sensation of your clothing against the back of your left thigh. But now that I've mentioned it, your brain has drawn your attention to it, raised it to the level of conscious perception, and you now perceive it as a result. This is an incredibly useful feature of your brain, because if you were forced to process all the information you receive during every second of every day, you would be so overwhelmed by sights, sounds, and feelings that you wouldn't be able to accomplish much.

This processing does take time. In fact, it can take up to about half a second for a given stimulus to reach the level of your conscious perception—in other words, for you to realize what's actually happening.

Your reflexes, however, respond much faster, in approximately 100 milliseconds, or one tenth of a second. This is why you're sometimes able to respond to things before you're even aware of what's happening. In certain situations (such as when there's a perceived threat) your brain is able to receive that information and direct your body away from the threat without you even being consciously aware of what's happening.

Interestingly, humans can actually improve the speed of their conscious perception with training. Now, as a lifelong fan of motor sports, I have to bring up the fascinating example of how Formula 1 drivers use this to their advantage. These elite racers can actually speed up (pun intended) their conscious perception to around 200 milliseconds, about twice as fast as the average person. This has nothing to do with talent or genetics—it's just from practice. As part of their job, F1 drivers undergo extensive neurological and reaction speed training—tapping lights, catching balls, and training in simulators for thousands of hours—to sharpen these systems which are crucial for race-winning, and potentially lifesaving, maneuvers.

This suggests that while their reflexes aren't necessarily faster than the average person, their conscious processing (AKA reaction times) has been dramatically enhanced through practice. Anecdotally, I've experienced a version of this myself. Even after a few days at racing school—a hobby of mine that I partake in several times a year—driving on normal streets feels like slow motion, and my overall driving has noticeably improved (just don't ask my wife). Imagine what *decades* of this training does for professional drivers!

You even have built-in reflexes that don't make it all the way up to your brain, such as when you step on a nail. That signal enters your spinal cord, then shoots right back out to pull one foot up (off the nail) and the other down toward earth to support your balance.

All this to say, your brain is an incredibly complicated system that in one way or another interacts with and ultimately affects every other part of your body, all the while integrating vast amounts of information from the outside world. If your neurons can no longer communicate with one another like they should, or if they begin dying at faster rates than normal, this can set off a cascade of events leading to much larger problems in the brain and the rest of the body.

Your brain does, however, have an incredible capacity to buffer problems and keep all systems working even when some things are going wrong at a cellular level. This is called your **cognitive reserve**, and while it is a useful feature, the tradeoff is that damage can accumulate undetected for years. This is partly why neurodegenerative diseases like Alzheimer's and Parkinson's disease are so hard to treat—by the time symptoms rear their ugly heads, it's often too late.

We do lose neurons as we age, and a certain amount of cell death is normal. The process of **pruning**, for example, is the programmed loss of excess neurons and synapses—a critically important part of how your brain developed in your early years to help reinforce important connections and omit others. But *premature* aging or death of neurons is not useful.

LEARNING AND MEMORY

Seeing as you're here to learn how to live a longer, healthier, and more impactful life, it would serve us well to discuss how learning actually works. This is one of the key systems to maintain as you age, and the lifestyle choices you make on a daily basis have a dramatic impact on your ability to preserve this part of your brain.

The ability to learn and retain memories is something we often take for granted. It's something most people don't ever even think about until they see it start to impact someone they love—at which point it becomes painfully obvious how important it is. One of the hardest parts of my job as a neurologist is watching families navigate their loved one's memory slipping away. I see this play out almost daily in hospitals across the country, and while you might think these conversations would blur together at a certain point, I can remember most of them clearly, which is a blessing and a curse.

Take Susan, for example. I can vividly remember Susan's pleasant smile as I walked into her room on the neurology ward one morning. When I asked her how her day was going, she responded cheerfully, "It's going very well, dear, how about you?"

Susan could readily tell me the names of her children, her husband, and perform all the complex motor tasks I routinely ask of my patients during their detailed neurological assessment, but the trouble arose when I asked her what day it was. Befuddled, Susan said, "I'm so sorry, dear—I don't know what day of the week it is. I just don't keep up with these things anymore."

When I asked her the month, I received the same response. Followed by the year, the President of the United States, and even where we were. She simply could not tell me the answers because she didn't know. I then asked her to remember and repeat the same three words that I ask all my patients: *ball, flag, tree*. Sadly, Susan failed this task, as well.

Knowing that we had already exhausted an otherwise thorough workup to explore any alternate explanation for her progressive memory loss over the past six months, I turned to Susan's daughter and said the painful words I've been forced to recite to the children of so many other patients, "I am so sorry to tell you this, but I believe your mother has Alzheimer's." It is the countless moments like these that ultimately drove me to write this book—so that you can hopefully avoid this future for yourself and find a better outcome.

Alzheimer's is a tragic example of what happens when we lose function in the learning and memory retention portions of our brain. This can also happen in other ways as we age and is part of what can be generally described as cognitive decline. However, both Alzheimer's and cognitive decline are largely preventable through lifestyle habits. (We'll discuss this more in depth later, but to be clear, less than 1 percent of Alzheimer's cases are genetic, whereas the vast majority are simply the result of molecular consequences that add up over a period of decades largely due to lifestyle habits.)

When you begin to understand the mechanisms behind learning and memory retention, you can see how certain interventions like sleep and simply staying mentally active can help preserve these parts of your brain and keep them functioning well into your later years. The more you can do to keep your brain healthy, the better your chances will be—not only for preventing neurologic diseases like Alzheimer's, but simply staying sharper for longer.

So, let's explore how this works.

THE HIPPOCAMPUS

When you encounter new information destined to end up as a memory, the first place it ends up is a little seahorse-shaped structure deep within the middle of your brain called the **hippocampus,** originally named from the Greek word for seahorse. (We technically have two hippocampi, one in each hemisphere of the brain.) The information at this point exists as what's called a **neural pattern**—a specific sequence of electrical activity between your neurons that can then be replayed. A loose analogy would be to think of this like a file on a hard drive, which at the end of the day is just a collection of electrical signals in binary code (ones and zeros). When your brain receives incoming information, it sends it to the hippocampus, which creates a temporary file that can then be recalled later.

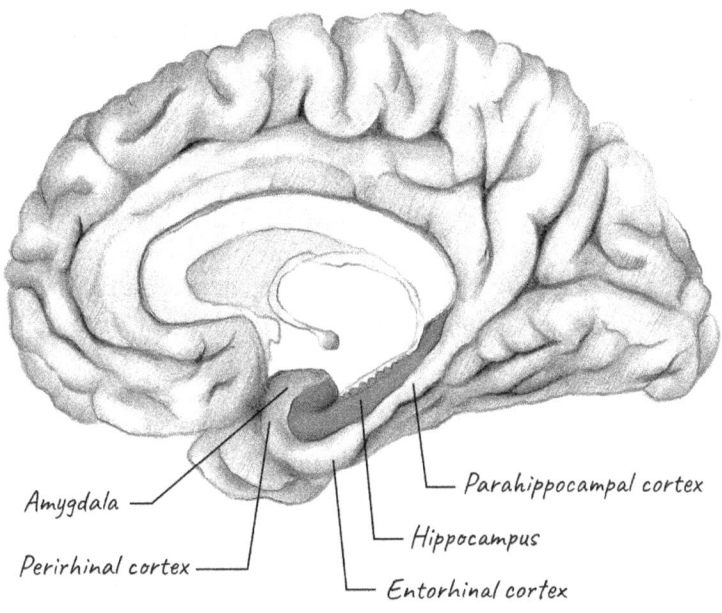

DIAGRAM 3: *The Hippocampus (and its location within the brain)*

This little structure is how you're able to recall what you had for breakfast this morning, the name of a new acquaintance, or even three simple words that a neurologist might ask. It's also one of the areas of the brain that is classically first affected by Alzheimer's, which is why Susan had so much trouble with my questions. The loss of short-term memory is a hallmark feature of Alzheimer's and eventually other forms of dementia.

The reason I referred to the "file" in the hippocampus as temporary is because the vast majority of your learning and the formation of long-term memory actually takes place while you sleep. During sleep, the hippocampus continuously replays those neural patterns associated with your newly-learned information. Thanks to neuroplasticity, the connections between your neurons in various regions of your brain then become strengthened, which makes it easier to access your new memories in the future.

This is why sleep is so important for memory retention and why pulling an all-nighter to study for a big exam is not ideal. Without sleep, your brain doesn't have the chance to actually form the connections required to represent all that new material you spent so much time cramming for—not to mention, your cognitive performance after a poor night's sleep is abysmal anyway, so there are two strikes. Assuming you have a somewhat decent grasp of the material to begin with, you'd be better off getting a good night's sleep than staying up all night so that you can better strengthen those new connections and recall the information the next day.

Now, these connections are only one piece of the puzzle. Your long-term memories are stored using a specific type of neuron called an **engram cell**, which becomes activated during a learning experience. Engram cells exist in various regions of your brain and store two types of long-term memory—conscious (explicit) and unconscious (implicit) memories.

Conscious memories are what most of your memories consist of. They represent things you can recall, such as the appearance of your childhood bedroom or the day you graduated college. These memories are largely stored in engram cells within the medial temporal lobes of your brain, right next to your hippocampus. If you put your fingers behind your ear and feel the little round bony protrusion there, that's your temporal bone. Just past that are your temporal lobes, and you have one on each side. So, when you read "your childhood bedroom" and pictured it in your mind, what really happened was the engram cells in your temporal lobe synchronously fired, allowing you to access that (hopefully) nostalgic image.

There are two types of conscious memory: **episodic** and **semantic**. Your **episodic memory** allows you to recall personal experiences, such as the details of your aunt's fiftieth birthday party that took place in your grandmother's living room. Your **semantic memory** allows you to recall basic facts or general knowledge independent of personal experience, such as knowing that Europe is a continent.

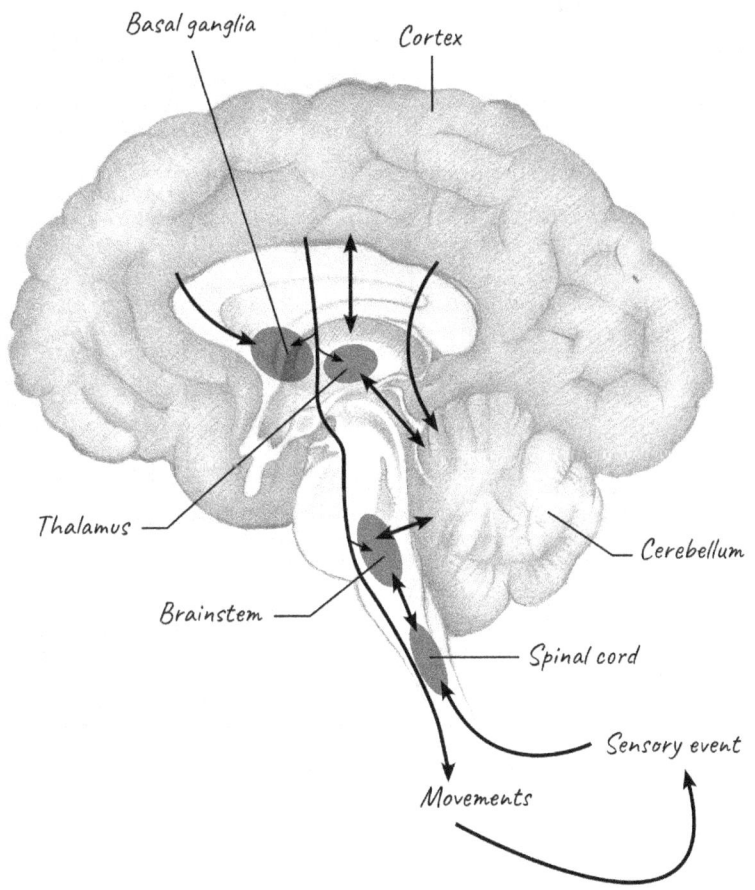

DIAGRAM 4: *BASAL GANGLIA & CEREBELLUM*
(Where unconscious memories are stored)

Unconscious memories are similar to what you might think of as "muscle memory." These memories are mostly related to how to do something, like how to serve a tennis ball or ride a bicycle, and they are stored in deeper structures of your brain such as the **basal ganglia** and **cerebellum**.

The **basal ganglia** are a group of structures deep in your brain that are heavily involved in fine-tuning motor movements. Your **cerebellum** sits in the back, lower part of your skull and is imperative for regulating balance and coordination. Given the fact that these areas store unconscious memories, this makes perfect sense. You rely heavily on unconscious memories when you walk, exercise, or perform your favorite hobby, and those memories are mostly stored in engram cells within the basal ganglia and cerebellum. The word *cerebellum* is also Latin for "little brain," as it looks almost like a smaller brain, so that's fun.

As you can see, your ability to learn and retain memories really just comes down to groups of cells working together in your brain. As you age, these cells can die off or become impaired, and you begin to lose your memory as a result. Therefore, the best way to preserve your memory is to simply slow the rate of cellular aging in your brain and keep those cells functioning well for as long as possible. This can be done through a variety of interventions that we'll discuss later, although sleep is perhaps one of the biggest levers.

Now, while we typically think of memory loss in terms of conscious memories, what about those unconscious memories? Given what we know of unconscious memories and their involvement in muscle memory, it would make sense that memory loss could also potentially affect your motor control—and it can. To understand this further, we'll need to take a quick look at how motor control works in the brain.

MOTOR CONTROL

Have you ever wondered how you're able to automatically control your body in precise fashion without actually thinking about it? For instance, when you walk, you're not forced to think, *Okay, now I need to pick my left foot up, move it forward, place it down. Now the right foot goes up....* instead, you just walk! That's because you have motor circuits in your brain that are dedicated to your **procedural memory**, which handles these things for you. This is incredibly important because it saves a massive amount of energy and frees up your brain to spend time thinking about more important matters.

Motor control relies on yet another incredible series of systems within our brains that most of us take for granted until something goes wrong. If your leg has ever fallen asleep after sitting for too long, you know what I'm talking about. Unfortunately, when things really go wrong here, they can be truly life-altering.

I recently cared for a patient named Paul who was just forty-three years old when a tiny blood vessel burst deep within his brain, causing a massive stroke. That ruptured vessel allowed a large volume of blood to accumulate in Paul's basal ganglia, the area we just touched on that helps to control movement. This specific type of stroke, known as a **hemorrhagic stroke**, was caused by long-standing, uncontrolled high blood pressure that had been slowly damaging Paul's blood vessels over time until, like a time bomb, the vessel finally gave way.

When this happened, it was like a light switch had been turned off, and Paul immediately lost all motor function on his left side. When we first met shortly thereafter, his left arm and leg were completely unresponsive—just dead weight. His stroke also affected the left side of his face, which caused his muscles and skin to droop and resulted in difficulty talking and eating.

> For those interested, the neurologic term for slurred speech is called **dysarthria.** Strokes can cause this or another type of speech problem called **aphasia,** where people speak in meaningful but short sentences, or produce fluent but nonsensical speech. To state the obvious, neither is good.

In addition to his physical weakness, Paul also lost some of his unconscious motor memories required to perform even basic tasks. For example, he had forgotten how to use utensils while eating. The most heartbreaking moments, however, were the times his son would try to call him. Even when he held his phone in his otherwise functional right hand, Paul could not remember how to operate it to answer his son's calls—he would just stare at this ringing device that had a picture and the name of his son flashing on the screen without the faintest idea of what to do. Fortunately, on more than one occasion I was able to answer or start a call for him, and as soon as he would see his son's or grandson's face on a live video chat, he would visibly perk up and smile (with the right side of his mouth, anyway).

Paul remained in the hospital for nearly four months, during which I observed him slowly recover some of the basic functions of the left side of his body. He was eventually transferred to a skilled nursing facility for long-term rehabilitation where he faced a serious uphill battle. I haven't seen him since, but given the extent of the damage he suffered, it's unlikely he will ever make a full recovery.

Perhaps most tragic of all is that this entire situation was largely preventable. Paul's stroke, like so many others, was the result of a series of long-standing, poorly managed chronic medical conditions that could have been prevented through the appropriate lifestyle interventions or even medication. Sadly, this is an incredibly common story I encounter day in and day out. This is the predictable result over time if you don't proactively maintain the systems in your body.

Tragedies aside, let's take a look at how this system is *supposed* to work. Your brain has three main networks that function together to control your movement: the motor cortex, the basal ganglia, and the cerebellum. When you decide you want to take that step forward, your brain first generates a signal in your **primary motor cortex**, which is a little strip of neurons on the outer part of your brain. That signal then gets relayed to your basal ganglia, which is that deeper set of structures we talked about previously. The basal ganglia essentially fine-tunes the signal, which then gets projected back to the motor cortex through the relay center in your brain, called the **thalamus**.

Similar to the hippocampi, you actually have two **motor cortices**, one on either side of your brain. Counterintuitively, the left side of your brain controls movement on the right side of your body, and vice versa. If you want to move your left foot, for example, the signal would start in your right primary motor cortex.

While this is happening, your cerebellum receives part of that initial crude signal and integrates it with incoming sensory information about where you are in space. The cerebellum also compares this new information with prior experiences and memories of that same movement, which further fine-tunes the message as it is simultaneously projected back up to the motor cortex. In one final step, this perfected signal then travels all the way down your spinal cord, where it jumps to a second nerve cell that has a long axon extending to your target muscle. When the signal finally arrives, it causes your muscle to contract, and you move.

And that's the simple version! Not to mention, this only partially illustrates the process for just *one* muscle contracting. Walking involves hundreds of muscles working in conjunction with one another, contracting and relaxing, to keep you moving and perfectly upright every single second of the day. Even standing still involves many muscle groups, which is why I'm a fan of standing desks—a simple intervention we'll address in Chapter 5.

While these systems are complex, they can operate quite well for most of your life when maintained properly. Think about how poorly your car's engine would run without regular oil changes or how limited your stopping power would be without new brake pads. Your body isn't terribly different, except rather than a major tune-up once every few years, the upkeep happens every minute of every day. As you'll discover in later chapters, your body is very good at repairing the cellular mechanisms inside your body, and this repair process is happening all the time.

Neurologists and neuroscientists often repeat the phrase "use it or lose it" because it is highly applicable to the brain ("neurons that fire together wire together" is another). This is generally true with respect to mental sharpness—the more you use your brain, the sharper you'll be for longer. The same can also be said for your movements—the more you engage in a particular behavior, the more efficient your brain becomes at performing it.

Critically, this works both ways. For example, if you don't use your muscles, they don't receive the stimulation they need and can become deconditioned. This can result in shrinking of the muscles or age-related muscle loss, which causes a whole host of other problems, including immobility.

An interesting example of the interrelatedness of these systems, according to a 2022 cohort study in *JAMA*, is that individuals who play racquet sports appear to live longer than those that don't, demonstrating about a 19 percent reduced risk of all-cause mortality. Running was a close second.

One hypothesis for why this might be the case is that both of these sports are very physically *and* mentally engaging. Racquetball players, for example, benefit from improved strength and cardiorespiratory fitness by playing the game, which helps to maintain strength, balance, flexibility, and metabolic health. They also exercise their visuospatial circuits necessary for depth perception, and their frontal and parietal lobes for planning their next move. This requires constant activation and training of motor circuits, keeping the brain active in multiple dimensions. The lack of contact is also a huge plus, which helps avoid unnecessary injury and inflammation in the brain. (It might just be worth trading your helmet for the court!)

The moral of the story is that training your brain can have a very real impact on your physical health, and vice versa. These systems are all interrelated, and ideally, we want to take actions that optimize and maintain the cellular mechanisms within our brains and throughout our bodies. This can create a cascade of positive effects, making a dramatic difference in your overall longevity.

A **visuospatial circuit** is a neural circuit in the brain responsible for processing visual and spatial information, enabling skills like spatial reasoning, navigation, and object recognition.

EMOTIONAL REGULATION

As we discussed in Chapter 1, your brain has a complex reward system that was originally designed to ensure your survival, but in the modern world no longer serves you as well as it once did. This system plays a pivotal role in your behavior and decision-making, but it's really just a tiny piece of the puzzle. Another unique feature of your brain is the ability to attach meaning to any given experience that presents itself, which can result in a variety of emotions. You have the ability to regulate your emotions, meaning you ultimately get to decide what meaning you attach to a given experience. This is an incredibly useful tool that can help improve the quality of your life.

For example, let's say you complete a difficult workout that produces the sensation of burning in your muscles. Your brain might initially interpret that as unpleasant or painful, but you can actually train yourself to reframe that sensation as something more enjoyable and thus experience a more positive emotion as a result. Critically, you'll then be more inclined to seek this experience again in the future. This phenomenon is known as **cognitive modulation**, and we'll cover more on how to use that to your advantage in Chapter 5.

The point is, you have the ability to reframe any situation to be subjectively positive, which can have a dramatic impact on your outlook and even your overall health! In fact, positive thinking has been shown in multiple studies to lower all-cause mortality.

Of the approximately 70,000 thoughts we have per day, nearly 80 percent of them are negative. This has been termed as our **negativity bias**, and like the basic reward system we discussed in Chapter 1, there were originally good evolutionary reasons for this. When your ancestors encountered a silhouette at dusk that *may have* resembled a lion, it would have been safest to simply assume it was dangerous and avoid it. As a result, they'd be much more likely to live another day, increase their chance of reproduction, and ultimately ensure the survival of their lineage.

Thanks to this inherited evolutionary negativity bias, we are literally wired to assume the worst, which might be great for avoiding lions, but not so much for conflicts in the break room. Over the past several hundred years, social life for us humans has changed quite a bit, but the circuits in our brain haven't had a chance to catch up yet because they don't evolve that quickly. When over-engaged, our negativity bias can result in pessimism, fixation on negative thoughts, decreased productivity, and at worst depression or even self-harm. Unfortunately, this pattern of thinking can actually get worse over time thanks to neuroplasticity (remember, "neurons that fire together wire together") because the more negative thoughts you have, the more likely you are to experience even more negative thoughts in the future.

The beauty is that it works in both directions: neuroplasticity can help you overcome your negativity bias and retrain yourself to reframe your thoughts toward the positive. In fact, an entire field, positive psychology, has been born in light of this discovery. Reinforcing and practicing positive thoughts can actually improve your health and even contribute to your longevity—and there's some very real evidence to back this up. For example, in 2024, a *JAMA* study looking at over 49,000 older female nurses found that those who reported regularly practicing gratitude had a 9 percent lower risk of dying from anything. How's that for mind over matter?

A major reason negative thoughts impact your health is that they can result in excess and unnecessary stress. Even low levels of chronic stress can place significant strain on your body, resulting in problems like high blood pressure, poor sleep, elevated blood sugar, heart disease, and even dementia. Therefore, anything you can do to alleviate excess stress can positively impact your health—and turning your negative thoughts into positive ones is a great way to do exactly that.

Research has also demonstrated that optimists generally find more success in life, whether that's through relationships or careers, meaning a positive outlook can certainly help you cement your legacy and live out your purpose. I also have to point out that, in addition to countless health benefits, having a positive outlook just makes life a whole lot more enjoyable!

The big lesson here is that most of the systems in your brain are highly trainable. You are in control, and just like you might train specific movements of your body to excel in a given sport, you can also train parts of your brain to function in ways that will not only help you accomplish your goals but improve your health in the process.

This brings us to our next topic, the idea of "willpower" and what it means for your health.

WILLPOWER

The **anterior midcingulate cortex (aMCC)** is a structure in your brain responsible for attention, impulse control, reward anticipation, movement, and emotion. It's also a perfect example of what happens when scientists run out of words to describe things, which is why I'll be referring to it as the aMCC.

This is yet another trainable part of your brain that sits deep within your frontal lobes. Interestingly, "super agers" (older adults who have aged well and retained increased cognitive ability) have been shown to have larger aMCCs than the average person. Why might that be? Well, a larger aMCC has been linked to maintaining a positive outlook and managing negative emotions such as stress or anxiety. It has also been demonstrated to increase in size with regular exercise, in particular by engaging in cognitively stimulating or difficult activities such as learning a new skill or completing a puzzle. The real trick to growing your aMCC, it seems, is continuously engaging in something you don't particularly enjoy doing.

The aMCC specifically grows when you push yourself beyond your comfort zone. The key insight here is that once an activity becomes easy or routine for you, it no longer stimulates growth. It's only by continuously challenging yourself with new and difficult tasks that this brain region continues to develop. The more you embrace challenge and discomfort, the bigger your aMCC will be.

Dr. Andrew Huberman, neuroscientist and host of the popular *Huberman Lab* podcast—as well as a major inspiration for me to write this book—has previously discussed the aMCC in the context of longevity. In a 2024 episode titled "How to Build Immense Inner Strength," he provides a case study on the aMCC by way of ultra-endurance athlete and former Navy SEAL, Chief Petty Officer David Goggins.

If you've never heard of David Goggins, this guy will blow your mind. He frequently accomplishes truly unbelievable feats of endurance, like running over 200 miles at a time *precisely because he hates running*. He describes these challenges as time spent in his "mental laboratory," where he likely stimulates significant aMCC growth by continuously pushing beyond what most would consider human limitations.

This concept of embracing difficulty extends well beyond extreme athletes. During my time as a Navy physician, I had the privilege of working with Navy SEALs and MARSOC Raiders, who were easily the most mentally resilient individuals I've ever encountered. The training program for Navy SEALs, called BUD/S (Basic Underwater Demolition/SEAL) school, is designed to test the absolute limits of human willpower over six grueling months. Most candidates who attempt this program are already in outstanding physical condition and have competitive athletic backgrounds, yet they still fail at a rate of over 80 percent.

The training involves intentionally planned and relentless physical, mental, and emotional stress including constant physical drills, cold water exposure, and extended sleep deprivation. Those who make it through have undoubtedly strengthened their aMCC, and their bodies, in the process.

What's the practical value in all this? The lesson isn't that you need to run ultramarathons or apply to become a Navy SEAL. Rather, it's that challenging yourself *is beneficial for your health*. In fact, the sensation of frustration is your brain's signal that it's learning something new. So, when you feel that familiar resistance to complete a difficult task, remember that's precisely where you need to be.

Embracing new challenges, whether it's learning a new skill, pushing yourself in a workout, or stepping outside your comfort zone in your career, creates lasting changes in your brain that correlate with improved longevity. And while correlation doesn't necessarily equal causation, the evidence suggests that people who continually challenge themselves tend to maintain better cognitive and physical function as they age.

THE HUMAN CONNECTION

You may have heard the phrase "humans are social creatures." I think it's safe to say this is largely accurate, especially when we look back on our history as a species. Your ancestors' safety depended on their ability to work well together. As a result, their social evolution resulted in cohesive, tight-knit groups to help ensure their survival by leveraging individual skills, abilities, and the collective wisdom of the group.

Fast forward a million years or so, and that same brain you inherited not only craves social connection but gives you the ability to cooperate amazingly well in groups of different sizes.

Consider for a moment that anywhere from 60,00–100,000 people pack into football stadiums across the country any given fall Sunday. Minus the occasional alcohol-induced scuffle, they all cooperate extremely well together. As a counterexample, imagine 80,000 chimpanzees packed into the Superdome in New Orleans—it would be absolute pandemonium, and they'd be swinging down Bourbon Street soon after they broke out.

This is largely because our brains reward us for engaging in social contact. For example, have you ever noticed how relaxed you feel after returning home to your partner (or dog) after a long trip, or even just a busy day at work? How about how much more comfortable you feel around your closest friends compared with a group of strangers? There's another neurochemical reason for this. When you experience the feeling of safety, such as when you embrace your partner in a hug, share the experience of bonding with another person, and yes, even petting your dog, your brain releases a neurotransmitter called oxytocin. This, along with dopamine, helps to reinforce those feelings and encourages you to seek similar experiences in the future.

Oxytocin allows you to feel more connected and secure within any relationship, whether that's with one person or a group. It can also increase your feelings of trust and empathy, which allows you to let your guard down and relax, thereby lowering your stress levels. We've already covered that lowering stress is incredibly beneficial for your health, but there are also some neuroprotective effects of oxytocin. For example, oxytocin can inhibit proinflammatory signaling molecules that can damage your neurons and cause neuroinflammation. That means oxytocin can lower inflammation in the brain, which is one of the four main contributors to premature aging and all-cause mortality that we'll cover in the next chapter.

The idea of human connection impacting longevity has become more popular in recent years, in part due to Dan Buettner's popular book and now Netflix miniseries, *The Blue Zones*. In his research, Buettner uncovered select communities around the world, now known as "Blue Zones," that appear to consistently harbor an unusually high number of people who live past one hundred years old. While his research uncovered several common factors among these populations like their adherence to a "Mediterranean diet" and incorporating daily movement into their lifestyle, perhaps one of the more interesting similarities is the presence of social connection.

In Okinawa, Japan, for example, people form social support groups called *moais*—small groups of friends who commit to supporting each other for life. In the Nicoya Peninsula of Costa Rica, multi-generational families often live together, with grandparents playing an active role in daily family life. And in Sardinia, Italy, elderly residents remain deeply integrated into their communities, regularly participating in local events and gatherings.

What sets these communities apart is how social connection is built into daily life. As we age, isolation becomes more common, raising stress, loneliness, and health risks. But in these places, interaction is a cultural norm, or a "positive default." People stay embedded in their communities, which gives them purpose, lowers stress, and provides support when life gets hard.

It's a simple but powerful lesson: If you want to live longer, stay connected. Even small rituals like a wave to your neighbor or a weekly game night could make a big difference.

LOOKING AHEAD

Your brain is the command center for everything you do, think, and feel, and without it, life as you know it would not exist. In this chapter, we explored three critical systems—learning and memory, motor control, and emotional regulation—that each play a vital role in maintaining both your lifespan and healthspan. While these systems are complex, the key takeaway is that you are in control of how well they function, and for how long. Proper maintenance over the course of decades, governed by the choices you make every day, can have a massive impact on where you end up later in life.

By understanding how these mechanisms work, even in simple terms, you can now begin to appreciate the why behind your intentional lifestyle choices. For example, let's assume you want to retain your cognitive function for as long as possible—which is probably not a stretch since this would give you a maximum opportunity to create your desired impact in service of your purpose. At first glance, something like exercise might not seem relevant to this goal, but given your now-cursory understanding of the mechanisms involved, it's easy to see how it does in fact have an impact.

First, exercise lowers your blood pressure over time, which means better blood flow to critical areas like your hippocampus and a lowered risk of stroke, which could cause irreparable damage to critical areas of your brain. (Consistent exercise has also been shown to actually grow your hippocampus by around 2–3 percent per year and can even *reverse* age-related memory loss!)

Second, exercise reduces stress and prevents inflammation in your body that can damage your neurons over time.

Third, it improves the quality of your sleep, which helps strengthen the neural pathways between your hippocampus and various brain networks, thereby enhancing your memory formation and retention.

Oh, and the act of exercise itself strengthens neural pathways in your basal ganglia through the repetition of movement, which keeps you strong, maintains your balance, and improves your cognitive function—all of which strongly correlate with a longer, more capable life.

Each of these mechanisms directly supports your memory retention and cognitive function in its own way, and they work together synergistically to create an even greater impact on your short-term performance and your long-term health. These are just some of the nearly endless reasons exercise has been consistently shown to be one of the most effective interventions for preventing cognitive decline, even if at first glance it might not seem directly related to brain function.

Remember, your brain and the rest of your body are intimately connected. What's good for one is generally good for the other. This is also why even seemingly minor changes to your lifestyle can be worth implementing—because they all add up and can collectively create a cascade of positive effects throughout your entire body, which compound over time.

Now, remember those questions I posed in the beginning of this chapter? Of course you do, thanks to your hippocampi! Here they are again. To put your newly acquired knowledge into practice, try to answer them in your own words—you'll find the answers on the next page for comparison.

1. How does sleep affect memory retention?
2. How can blood pressure impact your brain?
3. How could a problem in the "motor control" system in your brain also affect your memory retention?
4. Why is social activity beneficial for your brain?
5. Why might racquetball players live longer than others?
6. How can positive thinking impact your longevity?

ANSWER KEY

1. How does sleep affect memory retention?
During sleep, your hippocampus replays neural patterns from what you learned that day, strengthening connections between neurons and making memories more stable. This helps in the short term (like when studying for a test) but also helps prevent cognitive decline later in life.

2. How can blood pressure impact your brain?
Long-standing high blood pressure can damage the small blood vessels that supply crucial areas of your brain. When these blood vessels are compromised, brain cells don't get the blood flow they need to function properly, which can lead to serious problems, like various types of strokes, causing irreparable damage to key systems in the brain like motor control and memory retention.

3. How could a problem in the "motor control" system in your brain also affect your memory retention?
Brain systems are deeply interconnected. The basal ganglia controls movement but also stores unconscious memories. When one area is damaged, it typically affects multiple functions because these neural networks work together, not in isolation.

4. Why is social activity beneficial for your brain?
Social interaction triggers the release of oxytocin in your brain, which can lower stress and reduce inflammation—both key factors in longevity. This appears particularly true in Blue Zone communities, where people regularly live past one hundred and all have strong social connections.

5. Why might racquetball players live longer than others?

Racquet sports engage multiple brain systems simultaneously—motor control for movement, visuospatial circuits for depth perception, and planning centers for strategy. This combination of physical and mental engagement, plus cardiovascular benefits, strengthens neural connections throughout your brain—and as a group sport involves social connection.

6. How can positive thinking impact your longevity?

Your brain is wired to have a negativity bias. Persistently negative thoughts can raise your stress levels, which can put strain on various systems, especially your brain. Training yourself to think positively can therefore reduce stress and inflammation throughout your body. And thanks to neuroplasticity, the more you practice positive thinking, the stronger those neural pathways become.

KEY TAKEAWAYS

1. **Your brain is a collection of around 136–150 billion cells (86–100 billion of which are neurons) with trillions of connections between them.** All the functions of your brain from consciousness to motor control to memory retention are really just cells interacting with each other. Therefore, maintaining and optimizing brain health largely comes down to slowing cellular aging.

2. **Neurons that fire together wire together.** Thanks to neuroplasticity, the more you use the connections in your brain, the stronger they become. Consistent mental and physical activity, therefore, is key for healthy aging and retaining cognitive function.

3. **Brain health is physical health.** The systems in your brain and body are deeply interconnected, meaning what's good for one typically benefits the other. Mental stimulation, physical activity, social connection, and positive thinking are all proven ways to increase your lifespan and healthspan.

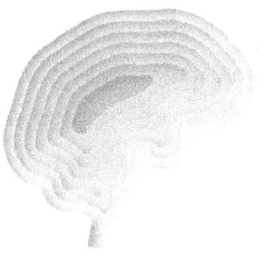

CHAPTER 3
THE PRIMARY THREATS

ONE OF THE GREATEST failures of Western medicine is its hyper-specialization. Physicians are trained to focus on increasingly narrow aspects of the body, often missing the bigger picture. In my field of neurology, over 92 percent of residents pursue a subspecialty, leading to a system where we no longer have general neurologists—only stroke doctors, headache doctors, epilepsy specialists, and so on. The same trend holds true across medicine: surgeons who only operate on hands, cardiologists who only do catheterizations, radiologists who interpret images from just one region of the body.

While this produces world-class experts, it leaves few physicians equipped to think holistically or practice true preventive care. Instead of understanding why diseases arise in the first place, we wait until a problem emerges and then intervene—often with a pill or a procedure. And the system rewards this reactive approach; providers are paid for treating disease, not preventing it.

But the truth is, many of the diseases that shorten lives or cause disability are deeply interconnected. The brain and body are not separate. The same root causes often underlie multiple conditions—and by addressing them early, we can prevent a wide range of issues before they start. That's the goal of this book.

I've grouped the major threats to your cognitive and physical longevity into four broad categories. While certainly not exhaustive, these represent some of the most common and preventable causes of early death and disability, and they're largely within your control:

1. Cardiovascular disease
2. Neuroinflammation
3. Neurodegenerative disease
4. Technostress

Because this book focuses on your cognitive as much as your physical health, I have intentionally not expanded upon several of the leading causes of death. But I would be remiss to not at least mention them for your reference, which is provided below. You should also know that the same mechanisms and interventions which apply to the four primary threats listed above also largely apply to lowering your risk of these other causes of death.

TOP TEN CAUSES OF DEATH IN THE UNITED STATES (ANNUALLY)

1. **Heart disease:** 699,671 deaths
2. **Cancer:** 608,371 deaths
3. **Unintentional injuries:** 226,999 deaths
4. **COVID-19:** 186,552 deaths
5. **Stroke:** 165,393 deaths
6. **Chronic lower respiratory diseases:** 147,382 deaths
7. **Alzheimer's disease:** 120,122 deaths
8. **Diabetes:** 101,209 deaths
9. **Kidney disease:** 57,937 deaths
10. **Liver disease:** 54,803 deaths

Back to our four primary threats. Let's take a quick look at each before we dive into the specifics.

Primary Threat #1: Cardiovascular Disease
The leading cause of death globally, cardiovascular disease affects your heart and the 60,000 miles of blood vessels in your body. Most often, it results from arteries becoming narrowed or blocked, leading to heart attacks, strokes, and other life-threatening conditions. But even before those events, restricted blood flow can quietly impair brain function and overall health.

Key interventions include:

- Regular aerobic exercise
- A heart-healthy, whole-food diet
- Managing blood pressure and stress
- Prioritizing high-quality sleep

Primary Threat #2: Neuroinflammation
This occurs when your brain's immune system becomes chronically overactivated. While acute inflammation is essential for healing, persistent inflammation can harm neurons and contribute to conditions like Long COVID, multiple sclerosis, and dementia. Neuroinflammation can be a silent threat, often progressing unnoticed until the damage is done.

Key interventions include:

- An anti-inflammatory diet rich in omega-3s and antioxidants
- Consistent exercise and quality sleep
- Stress reduction and toxin avoidance

Primary Threat #3: Neurodegenerative Disease

Conditions like Alzheimer's and Parkinson's involve the progressive loss of brain cells over time. While they may seem inevitable with age, many neurodegenerative conditions are the result of preventable lifestyle factors. Damage often begins years before the first symptom appears, which is why proactive brain health is so critical.

Key interventions include:

- Regular physical activity
- Mental stimulation and lifelong learning
- Strong social ties
- Achieving quality sleep and brain-healthy nutrition

Primary Threat #4: Technostress

Modern life bombards us with a level of information and overstimulation our brains weren't designed to handle. Constant alerts, emails, and digital noise create chronic stress and cognitive overload, accelerating aging across multiple systems. Like running a car engine at full throttle nonstop, this can wear us down over time.

Key interventions include:

- Setting tech boundaries and taking breaks
- Practicing mindfulness
- Prioritizing restorative sleep
- Moving your body regularly

Cardiovascular disease, neuroinflammation, neurodegenerative disease, and technostress represent the primary, preventable threats to your cognitive and physical longevity. While this is a highly simplified framework, most cases of premature death or disability trace back to one or more of these categories, which share common root causes and risk factors.

Each contains a range of specific conditions, like coronary artery disease or dementia, that may present differently but often arise from similar underlying mechanisms. By focusing on these shared origins, we can take proactive steps to protect our long-term health. In the sections ahead, we'll explore each of these threats in greater detail—starting with cardiovascular disease, the world's leading killer—and how targeted lifestyle changes can dramatically lower your risk of developing any one of them.

PRIMARY THREAT #1: CARDIOVASCULAR DISEASE

In hospitals, a code blue signifies the universal protocol for a patient presenting in cardiac arrest in need of immediate life-saving intervention—in other words, it's all hands-on deck because someone's heart has stopped, and they will die if they don't receive treatment as soon as possible. Without fail, I hear this multiple times a day when I'm working in the hospital, to the point where I don't even actively listen for them anymore because it would be too distracting. (It's also not my job to respond to them unless I'm the first doctor within arm's reach. Code stroke is different, which we'll cover momentarily.) Just in the time it took you to read this sentence, there were likely multiple code blues around the US, with each one indicating a life potentially cut short.

While I'm not part of the code blue team that typically deals with these situations, I've been involved in plenty of them. I can remember standing at the triage desk in the emergency department one afternoon, when I heard the call come in: "Yeah, we've got a forty-six-year-old male, no PMH, in v-fib...down time about twenty minutes per family, status-post two rounds of epi', two shocks, still no pulse, five minutes out..." I would soon find out that this "forty-six-year-old male" was Andy, a husband and father of three children in the prime of his career.

The paramedics came crashing through the doors of the emergency department, and we immediately sprang into action. I participated in a team of over a dozen physicians, nurses, respiratory therapists, pharmacists, and students all working frantically to save Andy's life. We took turns administering chest compressions, providing ventilations, delivering medications, and standing clear while over 200 joules of energy surged through Andy's lifeless body with each shock from the defibrillator—all in a valiant effort to restart his heart.

After thirty minutes, which felt like an eternity, no such attempt was successful. Andy was pronounced dead that afternoon after suffering a massive heart attack due to a blockage in one of the major arteries that supplied his heart. He had no preceding symptoms, and as the paramedics relayed in their call, "no PMH," or known past medical history. There were no warning signs.

Andy's story is unfortunately all too common. Cardiovascular disease claims approximately 50 million lives annually worldwide and as such accounts for roughly 30 percent of all deaths on the planet. And these aren't just statistics. Each one of these numbers represents a human life—someone's parent, spouse, sibling, or child. Each one of those people had hobbies, careers, goals, and dreams. What makes this even more tragic is that the vast majority of these deaths are *preventable*.

More than 523 million people worldwide are known to suffer from cardiovascular disease, representing a near doubling in prevalence over the past twenty years. Perhaps most concerning is that far too many people like Andy don't even know they have it until it's too late. The disease can progress silently for years before presenting as sudden cardiac death, like his did.

As mentioned in Chapter 1, cardiovascular disease is a uniquely human disease because unlike humans, wild animals stay consistently active, eat unprocessed foods, and don't experience the kind of chronic stress that plagues our modern society. While it might come as a shock to realize that even with all the incredible advancements we've made, wild animals are largely healthier than the average human, it does at least bring to light the inherently simple solution. Doing what your body was designed to do—staying active, eating healthily, and limiting stress—are all incredibly effective ways to avoid joining the 523 million people who face this problem.

At its core, cardiovascular disease describes a broad range of disorders affecting the heart, blood vessels, and brain. These disorders all share the same underlying mechanism. When the flow of blood to any part of your body is slowed or stopped, bad things happen, and they tend to happen quickly. For our purposes, the broad range of disorders that fall under this umbrella can be broken down into three main categories:

1. Ischemic heart disease
2. Cerebrovascular disease
3. Metabolic syndrome

The best way to understand cardiovascular disease as a whole is to take a closer look at each of these three categories. Let's start with the culprit of Andy's heart attack, ischemic heart disease.

ISCHEMIC HEART DISEASE

Ischemic heart disease, also known as coronary artery disease, occurs when the arteries that supply blood to the heart become narrowed or blocked due to a build-up of **arterial plaque**. Arterial plaque is typically composed of fatty deposits, cholesterol, calcium, and other substances—all things that accumulate over time primarily as a result of poor lifestyle habits.

As plaque builds up on the inner lining of your arteries, it can slow the rate of blood flow to your heart. When your vessels become narrowed enough, all it takes is for a piece of that plaque to rupture and form a clot, which can then block the vessel. At that point, oxygen, glucose, and other crucial nutrients are no longer able to reach the heart muscle and function immediately ceases.

This is what happened to Andy—the blood vessels supplying his heart had narrowed over time due to a buildup of plaque, eventually ruptured, and then a clot formed, completely blocking the vessel and triggering a **myocardial infarction**, also known as a heart attack.

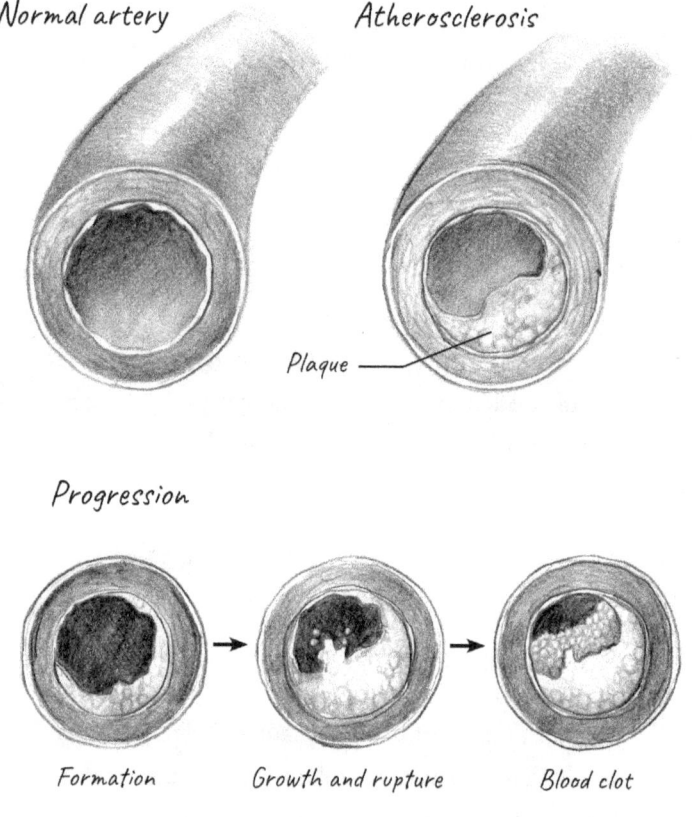

DIAGRAM 5: *Narrowed/Blocked Blood Vessel*

Perhaps the scariest fact about ischemic heart disease is that there are often *no preceding symptoms*. For a substantial number of the 50 million annual deaths from heart attacks, there's no warning sign and the first presentation of the disease is sudden cardiac death.

Fortunately, improved screening methods have become available (meaning heart disease is becoming easier to detect), although they are not universally available as of the time of writing. Advancing technologies like the Cleerly CT scan can provide a non-invasive way to determine the characteristics of arterial plaques and identify the likelihood of a blockage occurring. Regularly monitoring blood levels of Apolipoprotein-B ("Apo B"), Lipoprotein-A ("Lp(a)"), and Hemoglobin A1c ("HbA1c") can also provide increased predictive value relative to the standard annual lab markers your primary care physician might be monitoring. If you'd like to better understand your current level of risk, you might consider getting tested for those biomarkers among some of the others we discuss in Chapter 10.

That said, rather than taking the Western medicine approach of waiting until a problem occurs before trying to fix it, the far better approach would be to simply incorporate preventative measures into your lifestyle. In the case of ischemic heart disease and most of the conditions we'll be covering here, optimizing your exercise, diet, sleep, and stress levels are the primary interventions.

CEREBROVASCULAR DISEASE

Cerebrovascular disease, which most commonly manifests as a stroke, affects nearly 800,000 Americans each year. Like ischemic heart disease, cerebrovascular disease also occurs when blood flow is disrupted, but to the brain rather than the heart. The vast majority of strokes (approximately 87 percent) are caused by these blockages, while the remaining 13 percent occur from a ruptured blood vessel that causes increased bleeding within the brain, like Paul from the last chapter.

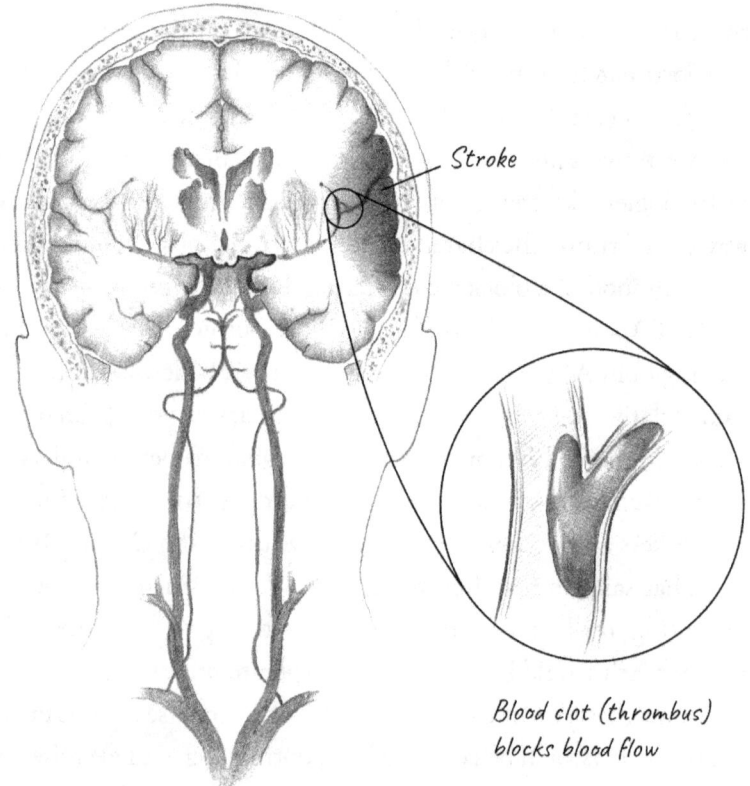

Blood clot (thrombus) blocks blood flow

DIAGRAM 6: *Stroke/Blockage cutting off blood supply to areas of the brain*

Your brain, as we know, receives around 20 percent of your body's total energy supply, which consists of primarily oxygen and glucose delivered via the bloodstream. This demand makes it particularly vulnerable to interruptions in blood flow—when the brain's blood supply is cut off, even briefly, symptoms occur within seconds. To put the severity of this into perspective, every minute even a small area of your brain doesn't receive blood flow equates to the loss of around 1.9

million neurons, 14 billion synapses, and 7.5 miles of axons. For this reason, there's only a narrow window of time—typically just a few hours—during which doctors can intervene to prevent permanent damage during an acute stroke.

Stroke symptoms can include weakness on one side of the body, difficulty speaking, loss of vision, confusion, or inability to walk.

When a stroke patient arrives at the hospital, there are a variety of methods we can use to remove the blockage in the brain to restore function, and the sooner we're able to do that, the better their chances are for a full recovery. That said, only 15–30 percent of stroke patients actually make it to the hospital within this critical time frame, which has been a major hurdle to effective care delivery for decades.

I can still remember one particular night (of many), when my pager bolted me upright at 2:00 a.m. with the message: "CODE STROKE: ETA 5 MIN." I made my way to the emergency department as Kathy was rushed inside.

At first glance, I could tell she was in serious trouble. She had gone to sleep only an hour beforehand, and her husband awoke to an unusual noise next to him. When he turned on his lamp, he saw that his wife couldn't talk or move the entire right side of her body, which prompted an immediate call to 911. I also noticed that her eyes were forced to her left and she was completely unaware of anything happening in the right side of her world.

Knowing that Kathy was likely in the middle of a massive stroke, we rushed her to the CT scanner where imaging confirmed a large clot lodged within her left middle cerebral artery, which supplies the majority of blood to the left hemisphere of the brain, the area responsible for all Kathy's symptoms. After quickly reviewing her chart and explaining the situation to her husband, he gave us permission to administer a powerful blood thinner known as tenecteplase, or TNK for short.

> **CT** stands for **computed tomography**, and a **CT scanner** is a device that uses multiple X-rays to create detailed, cross-sectional images of the body. This is how we pinpoint the exact location of blood clots in the brain when working with a stroke patient, the latter coming from a dedicated blood vessel imaging study known as a **CTA** or **CT angiogram**.

Blood thinners like TNK can quickly dissolve smaller clots and return blood flow to the brain in a matter of minutes, but they're often insufficient for larger clots. Although this was the fastest solution for Kathy, I knew it likely wouldn't be enough because her symptoms and imaging indicated a major blockage. I immediately called our interventional radiologist who prepared Kathy for a procedure called a mechanical thrombectomy, where a catheter was run through her femoral artery in her groin all the way up into her brain, and was used to manually retrieve her clot. The team extracted a nearly two-inch blood clot from her brain, which reopened the affected blood vessel and restored function to her right side. Miraculously, by the next morning, Kathy could walk and talk again.

While Kathy's case is a happy one, there are many who are not so lucky. For those who survive the initial event, a stroke can often have life-altering ramifications affecting everything from a person's movement to speech, vision, and more. This is why strokes are a leading cause of long-term disability and why avoiding strokes should obviously be a top priority for anyone looking to maximize their healthspan and lifespan.

When that initial treatment window is missed, a highly predictable series of events follows. Lack of blood flow means the neurons in the affected area of the brain do not receive the constant stream of nutrients they require and begin dying by the millions. After the stroke is "completed" (meaning the brain tissue downstream from the blockage is dead), in the weeks that follow the brain begins to heal and "remodel" itself, after which a scar is left, and function in that particular part of the brain is lost forever. Depending upon the location and degree of damage, function can be recoverable with intensive rehabilitation; however, there are many variables to this equation and complete success is by no means a guarantee.

The risk factors for stroke mirror those of heart disease: high blood pressure, elevated cholesterol, diabetes, obesity, smoking, and increased stress levels. This is no coincidence—these conditions all contribute to the same underlying mechanism, where blood flow is disrupted due to narrowing of the blood vessels that eventually result in blockages, just in a different part of the body.

METABOLIC SYNDROME

While not a disease itself, metabolic syndrome represents a cluster of interrelated conditions that can dramatically increase your risk of developing ischemic heart disease, cerebrovascular disease, type 2 diabetes, and other chronic health problems. This is why I've included it under the umbrella of cardiovascular disease—essentially, if you have metabolic syndrome, your chances of developing some form of cardiovascular disease are *very high*.

By definition, individuals with metabolic syndrome have three or more of the following conditions:

- High blood pressure
- High blood sugar
- Excess body fat around the waist
- Abnormal cholesterol levels
- Elevated triglycerides

What makes metabolic syndrome particularly alarming is its prevalence. An estimated 93 percent of Americans are considered "metabolically unhealthy," meaning that *nearly all of us* have at least one of these conditions knocking on the door. The vast majority of patients I see suffer from at least one, if not multiple, of these conditions—which is directly in line with the statistics. In most cases, these people end up in the hospital largely because of these underlying risk factors and the chronic diseases that arise as a result.

While I've easily seen thousands of people with metabolic syndrome, there's one patient that will always stick out in my mind, and whose story perfectly illustrates the far-reaching effects this condition can have on the body. During my time at the VA hospital in Washington, DC, I got the chance to meet Frank. Frank was a frequent flyer at the hospital, with a chart thicker than anyone I had ever seen. He was a Vietnam veteran who suffered from debilitating post-traumatic stress disorder (PTSD) that ultimately led to a handful of chronic health conditions. This is a situation that is unfortunately all too common with our nation's veterans, although Frank's case was a bit extreme.

Frank suffered from chronic stress as a result of his PTSD, which contributed to his development of high blood pressure. To cope with his stress, he often turned to sugary foods for comfort, which eventually led to diabetes. Largely fearful of leaving his apartment, a condition called **agoraphobia**, Frank became increasingly isolated and sedentary. His physical inactivity only worsened his weight gain and diabetes. As a result, he ended up losing both of his legs to infections several years apart, which stemmed from diabetic ulcers on his feet that he never felt or even knew he had.

Completely unaware of what was happening in his body, Frank continued to suffer through this lifestyle for the better part of two decades. His cholesterol levels crept up during this time, and in response, his body sounded the alarm by activating his immune system, placing him under a constant state of inflammation. Once this cascade began, it became increasingly difficult to stop. Frank kept returning to the hospital with stroke after stroke, which is how I eventually met him. On this particular admission, he was back for his *tenth* stroke.

> It is possible to have strokes that either cause no major problems or resolve themselves before significant problems occur. A **silent stroke** is a stroke that affects a small or redundant area of the brain, in which case you may never realize it has occurred. A **TIA,** or mini-stroke, is a fully reversible stroke that your body naturally resolves within a short time frame—typically seconds or minutes, although in some cases up to a few hours.
>
> (Not so) fun fact: I *often* see patients who have had multiple strokes without knowing it.

Frank had an advanced case of metabolic syndrome which impacted multiple organ systems, and was largely the result of mismanaged stress, mental health, and the resultant consumption of excess calories that were not offset by physical activity. We all know that consuming excess calories can lead to weight gain, but what's really going on under the surface when this happens? And why does this have such far-reaching impacts throughout our bodies?

When you take in excess calories, the energy balance in your body tips toward the "overnourished" or "constantly fed" state. When that happens, your body turns on genes that cause you to store that energy for a rainy day in anticipation of future need—largely by activating a pathway called mTOR, which we'll discuss in depth in Chapter 6. This was an incredibly useful feature that allowed your ancestors to go for days without food by storing enough energy in the form of fat while remaining physically active on their way to find their next meal, and you've inherited it.

In our modern society, however, where food is abundant and we rarely go for long periods of time without eating, this trait often does more harm than good—especially if we're not burning that stored energy through physical activity. When we continue to eat in this constantly fed state, our bodies keep storing that energy and we pack on the pounds. Consuming excess carbohydrates, which make up about half of what most Americans consume, is particularly problematic, as this can cause your pancreas to work overtime to try and keep your blood glucose levels in check. As a result, however, your cells become less responsive to insulin over time, which causes the problem to accelerate and results in premature cellular aging, which only leads to further problems, not to mention signals your body to store more energy.

In fact, most of that excess energy then gets stored as fat, much of which is deposited under your skin, where it becomes what's known as **subcutaneous fat**. Far more worrisome, however, is that increased sugar intake, decreased activity, increased stress, and less commonly some genetic predispositions can selectively increase storage of fat around your internal organs, which has been termed **visceral fat**. Visceral fat is particularly dangerous in that it elevates inflammation in the body. Over time this leads to chronic inflammation, altered communication between your cells, and epigenetic changes, all of which are key hallmarks of aging that we'll be covering in the next chapter. Life insurance companies even know this and will often reject applicants simply based on their waistline or because they have a "pear-shaped" body.

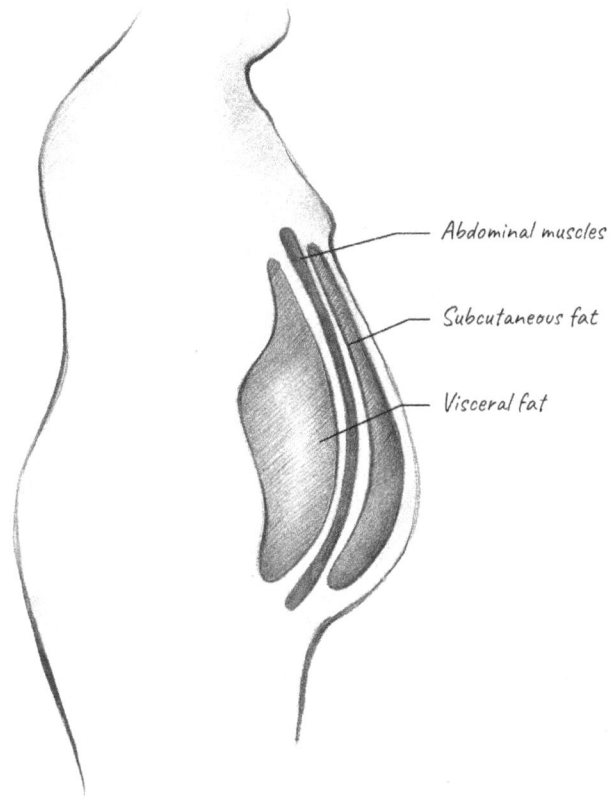

DIAGRAM 7: *Visceral Fat*

Frank's story is a perfect example of how these conditions rarely exist in isolation, but feed into and amplify one another. When you develop insulin resistance, for example, your body stops processing energy efficiently. This can lead to increased inflammation, which damages your blood vessels. This in turn contributes to plaque formation, which makes your arteries stiffer and raises blood pressure, which induces increased mechanical stress on your blood vessels. This causes even further damage, and eventually leads to problems like heart attacks, or in Frank's case, relentless strokes. This vicious cycle continues, with each condition making the others worse, and so on.

The silver lining, however, is that these mechanisms work both ways, and positive changes to your lifestyle can have a similar cascading effect in reverse. Like nearly all cardiovascular diseases, metabolic syndrome is entirely preventable in most cases. The same interventions that help to prevent heart disease and stroke—regular exercise, proper nutrition, stress management, and adequate sleep—can prevent or even reverse these precursors, especially when caught early.

PRIMARY THREAT #2: NEURODEGENERATIVE DISEASE

If you've ever watched a loved one suffer from a neurodegenerative disease, you understand the profound devastation these conditions bring to families. In the case of Alzheimer's in particular, while the person affected often remains largely unaware of their decline in the later stages—a small mercy, perhaps—their loved ones are forced to watch as someone dear to them slowly fades away, powerless to stop it.

These can show up in different ways. For some, it begins with small memory lapses—forgotten appointments, repeated stories, misplaced items. For others, it might start with subtle changes in movement—a slight tremor in the hand, handwriting becoming smaller and more cramped, movements becoming stiffer or slower than usual. But over time, these changes become more profound. The funny uncle known for his quick wit now struggles to follow conversations. The steady hands that once built furniture or created art begin to shake uncontrollably. The parent who never missed a game or recital struggles to remember their children's names. The spouse who loved to dance can barely walk without assistance.

If this feels heavy, it's because it *is* heavy. Having spent my career watching these diseases play out, I can tell you I wouldn't wish them upon my worst enemy. It doesn't matter how many times I see it unfold—it's painful every time.

The reality of neurodegenerative disease is difficult to confront, so we often push it to the back of our minds, treating it as some far-off possibility that we'll deal with later. Many assume it's simply inevitable, something that just happens to certain people as they age, outside of their control. But avoiding the topic or assuming it's inevitable is exactly the wrong approach. The truth is that barring rare exceptions, you have far more control than you might realize. There's mounting evidence that prevention is not only possible but probable; however, it has to start early—and that means confronting this reality today, no matter how uncomfortable it might be.

So, with that in mind, we first need to understand what we're dealing with. What exactly is neurodegenerative disease? At a high level, it's a blanket term used to describe a variety of conditions, most of which involve the progressive loss or withering away of brain cells, resulting in a gradual decline in brain function. Alzheimer's and Parkinson's are the two most common examples, although there are other, more rare conditions that fall under this umbrella, as well.

Though symptoms typically appear in elderly patients, neurological disease often starts much earlier. By the time symptoms emerge, significant damage has already occurred in the brain. And while there are treatments that can provide symptomatic relief or make life more comfortable for those affected, there are currently no known cures for any of these diseases.

I am hopeful and even confident there will be continued advances for available treatments in our future, but it's hard to say when those might appear. For now, your best hope by far is to minimize your risk of developing these conditions in the first place through intentional changes to your lifestyle. And because the changes that underlie these diseases typically develop for decades before the first symptom appears, it is absolutely critical to start as early as possible.

So, with that said, let's take a look at the two biggest neurodegenerative threats: Alzheimer's and Parkinson's.

ALZHEIMER'S

In Chapter 2, we met Susan, who struggled to remember basic facts like the day of the week or words I had said to her just moments earlier. Susan was experiencing the early stages of Alzheimer's, and she and her family had a long, arduous road ahead of them. While I didn't get a chance to follow Susan's care after she left the hospital, I can tell you almost exactly how her journey went. Because once diagnosed, Alzheimer's follows an extremely predictable pattern—one that I've seen thousands of times.

Another recent patient of mine, Mary, was on the other end of her Alzheimer's journey. She was in the late stages of the disease, and when I walked into her room she greeted me with a bright smile and a cheerful laugh. After allowing her to settle down, I told her "good morning" and extended my hand in greeting—a simple gesture I've performed countless times with patients over the years. What happened next was both fascinating and heartbreaking.

Mary studied my outstretched hand with the innocent curiosity of a child encountering a new object for the first time. She tilted her head to the left, running her fingers across mine to examine the texture of my skin. Apparently satisfied with this brief tactile exploration, she looked up at me, then returned her gaze to the empty wall in front of her, where it remained for the rest of our time together.

Her breakfast sat largely untouched on the bedside tray, most of it having found its way onto her hospital gown rather than into her mouth. When I asked her husband, who she hadn't recognized for well over a year now, how she was doing, he simply said, "Just another normal day, Doc."

Unlike Susan, who could still recall her children's names and perform basic tasks, Mary had not only forgotten how to eat and move properly, but she had forgotten who her family was and even her own name. This is the cruel reality of Alzheimer's—a gradual fading of one's essence that transforms a vibrant human being into someone nearly unrecognizable to those who know and love them.

Alzheimer's is a type of dementia—in fact the correct terminology for this particular diagnosis is "Alzheimer's disease" or "Alzheimer's-type dementia," but for the sake of brevity, we'll use the short version. For context, **dementia** is an umbrella term that refers to a progressive loss of intellectual and general cognitive function severe enough to interfere with daily life. There are many types of dementia, all of which affect approximately 50 million people globally, and this number is expected to triple to 150 million by 2050. Alzheimer's is estimated to account for approximately 70–80 percent of these cases, while the rest consist of various subsets of dementia. The specifics of each aren't terribly important to a non-neurologist, as they all eventually share the same basic hallmarks.

A primary feature of Alzheimer's is the progressive loss of neurons in the cerebral cortex, or gray matter, which is the outer layer of the brain responsible for the vast majority of our higher functioning. The hippocampus—that tiny seahorse-shaped structure from Chapter 2 that is responsible for much of your initial memory retention—is also classically affected early on, which is why short-term memory loss is often one of the first signs of Alzheimer's. As the disease progresses, further loss of neurons throughout the rest of the brain eventually leads to complete memory loss in addition to the loss of other critical functions.

One of the first known descriptions of the disease was published by German psychiatrist Dr. Alois Alzheimer, for whom the disease is named, in the early twentieth century. In 1901 he met a patient, Auguste Deter, who suffered from an unusual case of progressive memory loss and unexplained behavioral changes all too similar to what my patient Mary was experiencing.

When Ms. Deter passed away in 1906, Dr. Alzheimer performed an autopsy that revealed what he described as "a peculiar severe disease process of the cerebral cortex." He discovered microscopic changes in her brain that had never been previously documented—specifically, abnormal deposits of a protein called amyloid-beta, which had formed plaques between her neurons and neurofibrillary tangles within them, which were composed of a twisted-up protein called tau.

There are many different types of **plaque** in the body, and they all mostly refer to the buildup of debris. In this case, we're talking about **amyloid plaques**, which are sheets of beta-amyloid proteins in the brain, as opposed to the type of plaque formed in the arteries.

The accumulation of these abnormal proteins results in three major hallmarks of aging, namely a deficiency in proteostasis, impaired autophagy, and impaired mitophagy. We will cover all of these at length in the next chapter; however, you should know that **proteostasis** refers to the balance of normal protein function within the body, while **autophagy** is the process by which your body "recycles" the contents of your cells as they wear out. **Mitophagy**, which is also important, is essentially a subset of autophagy, the process by which your cells recycle their mitochondria after they die.

You may remember **mitochondria** as "the powerhouse of the cell" from your high school biology class, which is an apt description. Mitochondria are organelles found in most cells that generate energy through cellular respiration, converting nutrients and oxygen into **adenosine triphosphate (ATP)**, the main energy currency that fuels your body. There are hundreds or thousands of these in each of your cells, and preserving their health and function is essential for overall health.

In layman's terms, you can think of autophagy and mitophagy like recycling. When parts of your cell wear out, your body recycles them for reuse. This is an efficient system, but if there are problems, some of these misfolded and dysfunctional proteins from within your cells start to accumulate, which can result in a buildup of excess proteins amyloid and tau. Mitophagy is also particularly relevant because if this process isn't working correctly, that means your mitochondria can't provide sufficient energy to sustain normal function of your neurons, which is also thought to further increase the formation of amyloid beta and tau. While the early accumulation of these proteins doesn't appear to cause any immediate problems (because there are numerous asymptomatic people discovered to have them on autopsy), there's a certain threshold beyond which it appears to. We don't know exactly what that threshold is, and there's currently no great way to accurately determine the total amount of these proteins that have accumulated in someone's brain while they're alive—although several imaging modalities and blood tests for this exist. This is why once the symptoms appear, widespread damage has largely already occurred, and a person has reached a turning point from which there is likely no return. That is also why Alzheimer's is largely a clinical diagnosis, meaning it's based on symptoms—which, at this point, are well known.

When we dive further into the details, there are a few more mechanisms to consider. For one, damage to mitochondrial DNA is also thought to play a role in the development of Alzheimer's. When your mitochondrial DNA suffers damage, it can also lead to improper mitochondrial function, which increases **neuroinflammation**—an inflammatory reaction in the brain or spinal cord (which we'll talk about in greater detail soon). Increased neuroinflammation can then lead to **neuronal dysregulation**, or impaired functioning of your brain cells, which is also thought to contribute to the cascade of Alzheimer's. This is a big one, as chronic inflammation resulting from factors like obesity, visceral fat accumulation, insulin resistance, and more, is also known to cause neuroinflammation.

In addition to the conditions above, lack of exercise can also be a factor in the development of Alzheimer's. Remaining sedentary can decrease the maintenance and formation of new blood vessels in the brain and slow the production of two critically important signaling molecules, **brain-derived neurotrophic factor (BDNF)** and **nerve growth factor (NGF)**, which both stimulate neuronal health and are key to slowing brain aging. We'll go over exactly why in later chapters.

And finally, here's a blanket list of other known risk factors, *all of which are largely modifiable by optimizing your exercise, sleep, nutrition, supplementation, stress management, hormetic interventions, and general lifestyle choices*, which will be discussed in later chapters:

- Small vessel disease
- Atherosclerosis
- Stroke
- Metabolic dysfunction
- Dysfunction of the blood brain barrier
- Impaired blood flow regulation in the brain
- Impaired glymphatic function (the mechanism that removes waste from your brain)

Technically, there are some additional risk factors like cellular senescence, impaired energy balance, the failure of epigenetic mechanisms like DNA methylation, and an imbalanced gut microbiome. These will all be explained in further detail in the next chapter, as they have wide-reaching implications beyond Alzheimer's.

Although there's still some debate surrounding what ultimately causes the symptoms of Alzheimer's, the current evidence regarding prevention appears clear. The vast majority of cases appear to be the result of accumulated cellular damage over decades, with advanced age being the single greatest risk factor as most cases present at age sixty or older. How can you avoid this? Simple: don't let your brain get old! Another observation thankfully starting to gain more attention is the fact that Alzheimer's occurs *nearly twice as often* in women as it does in men. While the reasons remain unclear, with some early hypotheses pointing toward postmenopausal loss of estrogen accelerating the process of aging in female brains, this raises a serious problem that needs to be investigated.

Obviously, we can't slow down time; however, that does not mean Alzheimer's is inevitable or that avoiding it is simply a matter of luck. On the contrary, this is largely within your control, especially when you consider the fact that *less than 1 percent of Alzheimer's cases involve specific genetic mutations that cause early-onset Alzheimer's (the unlucky kind)*. The 1 percent statistic refers to people who have mutations in genes like amyloid precursor protein (APP) or presenilin-1 (PSEN1). These mutations result in early-onset Alzheimer's, which often presents itself before the age of sixty. While this is not a great situation for those affected, it is quite rare. It's also worth noting that it may be ameliorated or even eradicated with gene therapy in the not-too-distant future.

The other way genetics can affect Alzheimer's risk is through the APOE4 allele, which has been identified as the most common genetic risk factor for late-onset disease. Individuals with this allele have an increased risk of developing Alzheimer's, but they are by no means guaranteed to develop it. Carrying two copies of the allele increases your risk by about a factor of ten, and carrying one copy still increases your risk, just not as significantly. What this really tells us is that these individuals need to be particularly mindful of their lifestyle choices as this has an even more profound impact on their risk of developing this disease. Therefore, while genetics can play a role in the majority of cases, they're far less important than you might think.

So, what are those lifestyle changes? At the risk of sounding like a broken record, we'll be covering many of them in the later chapters that discuss specific interventions. However, given what we just discussed, you should already have a good idea—a proper nutrition plan, consistent exercise, managing your stress, and critically, getting enough high-quality sleep are likely the biggest modifiable factors. There are a handful of supplements that also affect brain health and are also worth considering, which we'll cover in Chapter 9. That said, there are a few interesting interventions specific to Alzheimer's that are worth discussing here too.

For instance, a Mediterranean diet has been shown to slow progression of or even decrease the incidence of Alzheimer's. A 2024 study published in the British journal *The Lancet* demonstrated that consuming just seven grams of olive oil per day reduced the incidence of dementia by as much as 28 percent. Similarly, another 2020 *Lancet* study indicated that avoiding head injury, high blood pressure, air pollution, excessive alcohol consumption, smoking (including second-hand smoke), obesity, physical inactivity, depression, and infrequent social contact can prevent or delay up to 40 percent of all dementia cases. Interestingly, correcting hearing loss with hearing aids appears to also reduce dementia risk, possibly related to the preserved stimulation of the temporal lobes via continued auditory input (which also house your hippocampi and are intimately involved in memory formation, if you recall).

The bulk of the literature, however, keeps returning to the importance of preserving your metabolic health. This makes perfect sense when we consider how central your mitochondria are to maintaining your energy balance and preventing the cascade of premature cellular aging. Therefore, maintaining an optimal energy balance through proper nutrition and exercise can help preserve healthy cellular function, potentially preventing the first domino from falling that could set off the cascade of age-related changes that ultimately increase your risk of developing dementia.

PARKINSON'S

When I was five years old, I didn't quite understand why my grandfather couldn't stand, play with me like my other grandparents, or even shave himself. One of my earliest memories is sitting with him in his kitchen, watching his home health aide administer his daily shave. I can remember it like it was yesterday. My grandfather sat in his wheelchair, nearly motionless, while his aide ran a safety razor across his cheek. I can picture his stoic expression and strong jawline, and I can still hear the sound of the blade across his skin.

By that point, he was confined to his wheelchair and barely able to speak. After my grandmother unfortunately passed away the following year, he was moved into a nursing home where he spent the last five years of his life slowly deteriorating and further succumbing to the inevitable grip of Parkinson's disease. I also remember his emaciated, lifeless body when my mother and I saw him the day he passed away, which saddens me to this day.

While I'll never know for certain, I suspect that decades of exposure to toxic heavy metals and organic solvents at the printing press he owned likely played a role in the development of his condition. Like many neurodegenerative diseases, Parkinson's not only shortened my grandfather's life; it robbed him of his famously vibrant humor and his ability to do all the things he loved.

While I didn't quite appreciate the gravity of the situation at the time, I certainly did when it happened to my uncle. As an adult, I watched the same story play out with my aunt's husband who was finally laid to rest in 2020 after nearly two decades of *his* battle with Parkinson's. I used to dread the phone calls with my aunt, a former (and incredible) cardiac nurse, as we would try our best to make sure his treatment regimen was optimized, which became more and more difficult with each passing year. In the years preceding and since, I have seen the same story unfold time and again with countless patients over the course of my medical training and in clinical practice.

Parkinson's disease is the second most common neurodegenerative disorder behind Alzheimer's, affecting nearly 7 million people worldwide, with increasing prevalence and an estimated global burden of over 14 million by 2040. It is a highly disabling disease that results in increased stiffness of the body, shaking or tremors, slowed movement, and difficulty walking, which as a syndrome is collectively referred to as "Parkinsonism." Over time, it can also affect other body systems that involve sleep, digestion, blood pressure, and memory.

Like Alzheimer's, age is the single most important risk factor for Parkinson's, with most cases presenting after age sixty-five. This is a topic we'll keep returning to, and for good reason. If we can slow down or even stop cellular aging altogether, this appears to go a long way in decreasing the incidence of the majority of chronic diseases we face, not to mention keeping you functioning at your best.

Genetic mutations that cause Parkinson's have been identified; however, they are present in less than 10 percent of all patients diagnosed, and it remains unclear to what degree they fully play a role in manifestation of symptoms. Environment and lifestyle are thus believed to have a much greater influence on the risk of developing Parkinson's than any genetic predisposition. Pesticide exposure has emerged as the highest environmental risk factor in multiple studies, with those living in rural areas and consuming well water appearing to be at the highest risk. Exposure to air pollution, heavy metals, hydrocarbon solvents such as trichloroethylene, high dietary iron, and low vitamin D, among others, have also been correlated with increased risk of developing the disease.

While the exact cause of Parkinson's isn't fully understood, we know that it shares a similar hallmark to Alzheimer's. Just as Alzheimer's patients are found to have an overaccumulation of abnormal proteins in their brain, Parkinson's patients are found to have an overaccumulation of a protein called alpha-synuclein within their neurons. After this buildup occurs, it can trigger premature programmed cell death and even spread to adjacent, healthy cells, ultimately leading to their death. There are several theories as to why this happens, but to make a long story short, impaired metabolic health and premature aging of cells in the brain likely play a central role.

One way this is thought to happen is that when autophagy (if you recall, your cells' major recycling process) malfunctions, it can lead to the accumulation of a misfolded version of alpha-synuclein that accumulates over time within the neurons. This disruption of autophagy and loss of proteostasis—the ability for proteins to function normally—ultimately lead to neuronal dysfunction and eventually widespread cell death.

Like Alzheimer's, mitochondrial dysfunction also appears to be relevant in the development of Parkinson's. In the disease, mitochondrial activity is substantially reduced within dopaminergic cells. In addition to the reward circuits we discussed in Chapter 2, dopamine also plays a critical role in movement—too much can lead to excessive movement and too little to decreased movement and stiffness, which is what is seen in Parkinson's. Consequently, when enough of these cells are lost, symptoms begin to show up.

> **Dopaminergic cells**, the neurons that produce and release dopamine, are primarily located within the midbrain, in an area called the **substantia nigra,** Latin for "black substance," and named for its dark appearance.

Long before the appearance of clinical symptoms, other changes in the brain and the body are known to take place. By the time the first symptoms of Parkinson's emerge, well over 60 percent of these dopaminergic cells within the midbrain have already died, implying that, like Alzheimer's, there's a similar threshold that our brains can accommodate—but only for so long.

So, how does this cascade of events start in the first place? While that continues to be investigated and largely a matter of debate, there is some evidence that Parkinson's may actually start in the gut and not the brain itself! This idea was initially proposed by neuropathologist Heiko Braak, who observed alpha-synuclein deposits in the **enteric nervous system**—the network of nerves that control your digestive system—and suggested that an external pathogen may enter the nasal cavity, which is then swallowed, arrives in the gut, and ultimately reaches the brain via the vagus nerve.

While this model has come under scrutiny for a variety of reasons, we now know the **gut-brain axis** (the connection between your gut and brain) appears to play an important role in much of your body's immune function, mood and behavior regulation, and the production of neurotransmitters, all of which raise interesting considerations surrounding its involvement in Parkinson's.

There are several known symptoms that can manifest in the body long before the development of Parkinson's, some of which support the Braak hypothesis. Many of these are also nonspecific, meaning if you happen to experience them, there's a high likelihood that it's due to something else and not Parkinson's. These are, in no particular order:

- Decreased sense of smell
- REM Behavior Disorder (where patients act out their dreams in their sleep)
- Changes in digestion and blood pressure
- Depression
- Changes in bladder and reproductive function

So how can you lower your risk of developing of Parkinson's later in life? Once again, optimizing your lifestyle appears paramount to lowering your risk. Avoiding the environmental exposures referenced above appears to be a significant intervention. Achieving regular exercise, ensuring an anti-inflammatory diet high in polyphenols and antioxidants, avoiding traumatic brain injuries (largely suspected to be responsible for Muhammad Ali's diagnosis), and avoiding metabolic disease like diabetes all appear to lower risk.

Like Alzheimer's, there are also a few other unique interventions that have been shown to make a difference. Increased caffeine intake appears to be neuroprotective, with some evidence potentially pointing to the benefits of polyphenols serving as antioxidants in freshly ground black coffee. Interestingly, cigarette smoking has also consistently demonstrated a decreased risk in developing Parkinson's. This has suggested a potential neuroprotective effect of nicotine; however, to be clear, *smoking should be avoided at all costs* given the endless detrimental risks associated with it.

Neuroprotective is a blanket term that refers to any strategy or intervention that protects neurons from damage or degeneration.

As we close out our exploration of Alzheimer's and Parkinson's, it's worth noting that there are a handful of other less common neurodegenerative conditions. These include other types of dementia like the tauopathies, synucleinopathies, as well as even more rare conditions like Huntington's Disease, spinal muscular atrophy (SMA), and Amyotrophic Lateral Sclerosis (ALS). For our purposes, it's not worth diving into further detail, as they affect a very small subset of individuals and share similar underlying pathological traits to Alzheimer's and Parkinson's.

PRIMARY THREAT #3: NEUROINFLAMMATION

When I first met Cindy, I knew something wasn't adding up. While her symptoms initially suggested a stroke, her progressively deteriorating condition told a different story—one that would reveal how your brain's own immune response can sometimes become your enemy.

I was consulted after Cindy had been diagnosed with what appeared to be a stroke affecting her ability to speak. Her CT scan showed an abnormal area in her left temporal lobe (that part of your brain we discussed in Chapter 2 that sits just behind your ear), which explained her speech difficulties. What deeply troubled me, however, was that she was getting measurably worse each day, which is highly unusual for a typical stroke.

Cindy had woken up on a Monday with mild confusion, and her doctor had sent her home with a prescription for bed rest. By Wednesday, she was struggling more with her words, leading to her hospitalization and initial stroke diagnosis. But given her story and worsening condition, I suspected we were dealing with a different kind of brain emergency. I immediately ordered a high-dose antiviral medication and requested an urgent MRI and lumbar puncture (to analyze her cerebrospinal fluid) to better understand what was happening in her brain. Before I could even finish making those arrangements, I received an emergency page that Cindy was in the middle of a continuous seizure.

What followed was a coordinated emergency response as we worked quickly to protect her brain. We administered anti-seizure medications while the critical care team ensured her brain remained oxygenated. What we soon discovered was that Cindy wasn't having a stroke at all—her brain was under attack from within, experiencing massive inflammation triggered by a viral infection.

Cindy survived her initial crisis after two weeks in intensive care, during which time her brain infection was thankfully treated, but her journey was far from over. For the next six months, her immune system would periodically flood her brain with inflammatory molecules and immune cells, a condition known as **autoimmune encephalitis**. Each of these episodes required intensive treatment to calm her immune response in an attempt restore her brain function. This is neuroinflammation in its most dramatic form—when the brain's immune response becomes overactive, ultimately causing more harm than the initial threat it's trying to fight.

While Cindy's case represents an acute and severe form of neuroinflammation, this process can manifest in many ways. Sometimes it develops silently over years; other times it appears suddenly and dramatically and can cause a host of problems.

Another example is **multiple sclerosis (MS)**, which is thought to be caused by excess neuroinflammation. MS is a potentially disabling inflammatory disorder that involves disruption of the axons in the brain and spinal cord, although in recent years has also been known to affect the cortex, as well (where most of your neurons reside). While the exact cause of MS is still largely unknown, there are many clues pointing to the triggers of this type of neuroinflammation. Low levels of vitamin D, smoking, obesity, and having had mono (mononucleosis) as a child or teenager are all known risk factors. What do all of those have in common? Inflammation. And the effective treatments? All centered around lowering inflammation.

Neuroinflammation is also a factor in traumatic brain injuries, certain psychiatric conditions, and even Long COVID. Just like many of the conditions within the cardiovascular umbrella revolve around the same mechanism—the slowing or blocking of blood flow—all these conditions revolve around the same basic mechanism of neuroinflammation, which ultimately damages healthy brain tissue.

Understanding neuroinflammation is crucial because it doesn't just involve acute conditions like Cindy's. Chronic, low-level inflammation in the brain has been increasingly recognized as a key risk factor in various neurological conditions, including many that we once thought were simply inevitable parts of aging. In addition to those previously discussed, neuroinflammation is also thought to be involved in neuropsychiatric conditions such as major depressive disorder, schizophrenia, and psychosis, as well as neurodegenerative conditions like Alzheimer's, Parkinson's, and likely others.

The factors that contribute to neuroinflammation are actually quite similar to those that affect cardiovascular disease. In somewhat of an oversimplification, people who develop many of the chronic conditions we've previously discussed are at risk of experiencing low levels of chronic inflammation throughout their body, including the brain. Your body essentially knows that something is wrong, and it tries to fight back by activating your immune system. The problem is that it's impossible for your body to heal its way out of this, which can lead to chronic inflammation that prematurely ages your cells and damages various organ systems, a process termed **inflammaging**. Once again, this also means the same lifestyle choices we've discussed—exercise habits, nutrition, stress management, and sleep—play a crucial role in lowering neuroinflammation too (surprise).

There are, however, two unique risk factors for neuroinflammation that are worth discussing: **Long COVID** and **traumatic brain injuries**. Both of these conditions have taught us important lessons about how inflammation can affect our brains, and more importantly, how we can protect ourselves. Much of the evidence to support this has only surfaced in recent years, so I suspect we'll be hearing a lot more about neuroinflammation in the years to come—including additional risk factors and interventions to consider.

LONG COVID

Like most people, the COVID pandemic caught me completely off guard. I can still remember watching the sunrise on the Hudson River, the cold wind stinging my face as I stood in formation on the flight deck of the USNS Comfort as a young Navy lieutenant. It was April 2020, and I was one of several thousand troops deployed to what would become one of the worst epicenters of the COVID-19 pandemic. If you remember seeing images of that massive white hospital ship sailing past the Statue of Liberty on the news, that's the one I was on. And while I knew this was serious, I was then clueless about the profound effect it would have on all our lives for years to come.

Armed with nothing more than a face mask and the will to help, we faced an invisible enemy about which we knew almost nothing and against which we had no effective treatment. What followed was one of the most challenging experiences of my medical career. For six weeks, we watched helplessly as people died at an unprecedented rate, separated from our families, all while fearing for our own lives.

To put the severity into perspective, there was one gangplank on or off the ship, and I would have to wait daily to board as dead bodies were carried off. It got so bad that all the morgues in New York City eventually filled and civilians were showing up in personal vehicles, loading their trunks with bodies, then driving them out to Hart Island, where inmates from Rikers Island prison were burying them by the thousands. To say this was surreal would be the understatement of my life—it literally felt like a warzone. I was also tasked with the heartbreaking collateral duty of calling the family members of patients who didn't make it, as no one was allowed to board the ship to tell their loved one goodbye. This was the darkest moment in my career and one I am glad to be past.

After that nightmare of a deployment, I returned to my duties at

Naval Medical Center Camp Lejeune, where another peculiar syndrome began to emerge. Every week, my clinic schedule showed an increasing number of new referrals for lost sense of smell, brain fog, or memory loss. While I was accustomed to seeing these symptoms in older adults for one reason or another, this was different—these were otherwise healthy twenty-year-old individuals. Kids!

These service members' primary care providers had already conducted thorough evaluations but found nothing obviously wrong. My subsequent neurological assessments also yielded few clues beyond their persistent symptoms, which were significant enough to impact their ability to remain combat-effective—a critical requirement for any US Marine or sailor.

These cases, along with similar reports worldwide, would eventually become known as Long COVID. While we're still learning about the exact mechanisms involved, there's significant evidence that between 10–35 percent of COVID survivors report ongoing symptoms, including fatigue, cognitive difficulties, depression, anxiety, and memory problems lasting more than twelve weeks after their initial infection. While theories vary, neuroinflammation is thought to be the likely culprit.

What's particularly interesting is that people with a pre-existing diagnosis of metabolic syndrome tend to be more susceptible to and have some of the worst outcomes with long-COVID. Given our basic understanding of the mechanisms involved, it's easy to see why this might be the case. COVID is a particularly pro-inflammatory viral illness, meaning it causes more inflammation in the body than many others tend to. As we know, individuals with metabolic syndrome already experience some degree of chronic inflammation, so when they contract COVID, it's like gasoline on a fire. In response to the infection, inflammation spikes even further—and if it becomes dangerously high, it can result in heart attacks, strokes, clots in the deep veins of the body, or a life-threatening fluid buildup in the lungs. For reasons that are still not entirely understood, the brain appears particularly susceptible to persistent low-grade inflammation afterward, resulting in the symptoms mentioned above.

So, what can you do about this? The first and most obvious solution if you feel you are at high risk or have any pre-existing risk factors would be to get the COVID vaccine and maintain immunity through regular boosters. If you've made it this far, I have a hunch that you believe in the science behind vaccines like I do—not just for COVID but the array of conditions that have been eradicated over the past century due to their development. Vaccines are highly effective, the side effects for most people are negligible, and they can mean the difference between life and death for not only you, but others in your life—and I'll leave it at that.

There are some other treatments that have also shown to be effective, like low-frequency repetitive transcranial magnetic stimulation. That jumble of words basically means using a machine to direct magnetic current to different parts of the brain, using certain frequencies to "rewire" circuits and enhance neuroplasticity. In addition to alleviating the symptoms of Long COVID, this technology has also been shown to improve mood and help with depression.

Hyperbaric oxygen therapy may also be effective. Forty minutes of 100 percent oxygen at a pressure of greater than 1 atmosphere has shown improvement in cognitive symptoms from Long COVID. This has been thought to enhance neuroplasticity as well, and potentially improve stem cell regeneration within the brain.

Another interesting development is maintaining adequate levels of vitamin D, which has been correlated with lower mortality in the setting of COVID infection. In addition to maintaining bone health, vitamin D plays a vital role in immune system function. It is also thought to lower inflammation and oxidative stress in the brain in addition to regulating nerve growth factors responsible for brain health. If the theory of neuroinflammation in long-COVID is in fact correct, these mechanisms seem plausible.

Oxidative stress occurs when there is an increased production of free radicals due to an imbalance of oxygen in your cells, which causes increased cellular damage. In other words, having too much free radical production without the antioxidants to neutralize them can be harmful.

That said, there are many ways you can lower inflammation in your body through a variety of lifestyle interventions. Improving your sleep, having a sound nutrition and exercise plan, lowering stress, improving insulin sensitivity, curbing obesity, and avoiding anything that increases oxidative stress within your body, like smoking, are all effective interventions. Hopefully, this is starting to sound familiar.

TRAUMATIC BRAIN INJURY

A traumatic brain injury, or TBI, is defined as an injury caused by an external force such as a blow to the head, penetration by a foreign object, or a blast force that alters brain function. It is a leading cause of death and disability in people under forty-five, and something I unfortunately encountered regularly in my Navy career, as TBIs occur at a much higher frequency among active duty service members than civilians.

When you suffer trauma or injury to any part of your body, the healing process follows a predictable pattern. Your body responds by triggering inflammation in and around the affected area, which is why you typically experience swelling, redness, warmth, and pain after an injury—all cardinal signs of inflammation. In the short term, this is normal. It is how your body delivers the necessary cells, proteins, and nutrients for your injury to heal. Your brain follows this same basic principle when it experiences trauma too, but with a few critical differences.

For one, your brain tissue is very fragile and even a relatively mild trauma can result in bruising of your brain, tearing of brain tissue, injury to axons, and even bleeding inside your skull. All of this can happen as an immediate result of injury. However, in the ensuing days and weeks, inflammation takes over. While necessary to help your brain heal, when overactivated, it can result in chronic inflammation, which over time can cause widespread damage. It's a double-edged sword.

At a cellular level, this process triggers the release of excess pro-inflammatory cytokines. **Cytokines** are signaling molecules that you'll hear me talk about in many other places, and they are a crucial part of how your cells talk to each other. There are different kinds of cytokines, like **anti-inflammatory cytokines** (which lower inflammation) or **pro-inflammatory cytokines** (which cause inflammation). At normal levels, these are necessary, but if too many of the wrong kind are released, it can cause problems. In this case, too many pro-inflammatory cytokines are released, which can impair healthy brain function, healing, and even induce cell death if left unchecked.

This can also result in over-excitation of your neurons (which is not good, as too much or too little neuronal activity is bad—for an example of too little activity, just turn on the nightly news), increased oxidative stress, brain swelling, and disruption of the blood-brain barrier. All of this can result in further injury and the death of more neurons, which can result in loss of normal function. Chronic neuroinflammation can result in a cascade of negative effects that can impact everything from your memory to your ability to regulate emotions or even move normally.

> The **blood-brain barrier** is a protective, semi-permeable membrane that lines the inner surfaces of blood vessels in the brain, acting as a filter to regulate what substances can enter and exit the brain, protecting it from encountering harmful substances while allowing essential nutrients to pass through.

There are three primary levels of severity when it comes to TBIs: mild, moderate, and severe. Mild cases are referred to as concussions and are typically caused by non-penetrating head trauma, whereas moderate to severe TBIs involve more extensive damage to the brain and typically require complex medical intervention and management. That said, *any* form of TBI is a cause for concern, even if it doesn't present immediate symptoms. Recent research has also shown that it's not just the big hits we need to worry about.

When most people think about TBIs in sports, for example, they might think of two football players running at each other full speed, causing a massive collision. While linebackers and safeties are absolutely at risk for TBI, perhaps surprisingly, offensive and defensive linemen tend to have more long-term problems than many of the other positions. The reason is that while safeties and receivers take massive hits that make highlight reels, linemen experience dozens of smaller impacts per game, during virtually every play. These repetitive small collisions, which might seem insignificant in isolation, have now been shown to cause significant damage to the brain over time.

This discovery has changed how we think about brain injuries. We now understand that neuroinflammation can result not just from single traumatic events, but from the cumulative effect of multiple smaller impacts over long periods. This is particularly concerning because these minor impacts might not produce any immediate symptoms, making them easy to dismiss or ignore.

In fact, when looking at autopsy studies of former football players, reported concussions did not correlate with chronic changes found in their brain (changes which looked remarkably like Alzheimer's). In other words, the concussions weren't the only problem—it was the repeated smaller events over time. **CTE**, short for **chronic traumatic encephalopathy**, is the medical term used to describe this phenomenon.

Perhaps even more surprising is that it doesn't even take direct physical contact to incite a TBI. I mentioned that a blast force (such as an adjacent explosion a soldier might be exposed to) can be sufficient; however, it can even come from something far more innocuous. I have treated patients who have fallen on ice or from a bicycle and landed on their tailbone or an outstretched limb and suffered a clear post-concussive syndrome, which can only result from a TBI.

If you ever experience concussion symptoms, take them seriously—seek professional medical care and do your best to avoid further brain injuries. If you happen to play any contact sports, be sure to wear a helmet, and from the perspective of ensuring optimal brain health, you may want to consider a different sport with lower risk for contact.

Parents may also want to be careful enrolling their children in contact sports, as injury and neuroinflammation can also have a significant effect on developing brains. Regardless, the level of risk you are willing to tolerate is up to you—but whatever you can do to avoid minimizing your exposure to head injury will certainly be helpful.

PRIMARY THREAT #4: TECHNOSTRESS

Our final threat is something that affects the vast majority of people in our world today. So, rather than telling you a story about some patient of mine, I think it's time to turn the tables and hear your story.

Do you ever...
- Feel like you have too much to do?
- Feel like you spend too much time in front of a screen?
- Feel overloaded with the sheer amount of information thrown at you every day?
- Worry about looming deadlines or feel stressed thinking about how on earth you'll get all this "stuff" done?
- Suffer from decision paralysis, not knowing what to do given all the options at your disposal?

Chances are you said yes to at least one, if not all, of those questions. If you didn't, congratulations! You've successfully avoided one of the greatest pitfalls of modern society.

In Chapter 1, we talked about how your brain's inherited reward system has not yet caught up to modern times. Well, at a higher level, your brain is simply not designed to handle the constant stream of information that is thrown at you every day. Never before in human history have we been forced to consume this excessive volume of information, meaning your brain has not had sufficient time to evolve to accommodate these demands. Your brain is a processor, as you might recall, and it is being almost constantly overloaded. Think about how slowly your computer runs with multiple programs open and without a good reboot from time to time. Generally speaking, you aren't all that different.

For tens of thousands of years, your ancestors evolved with minimal exposure to information. They communicated about basic topics with words, gestures, and primitive tools. They had few choices to make, and their time was largely spent completing simple, repetitive tasks. They spent their days hunting, farming, caring for children, and building primitive shelters. They went to sleep when the sun went down and awoke when it rose. They ate what they farmed, gathered, caught, or hunted.

Over the past century and the past few decades in particular, technology has accelerated at an exponential rate, resulting in a constant and ever-accelerating influx of increasingly complex information. Smartphones, social media feeds, streaming services, and AI-generated content are inundating us with fragmented, emotionally charged, and largely notification-driven information—much of which is unsolicited or passively consumed. A huge portion of our population now spends a majority of their day staring at a box that shines artificial light into their eyes, conveying more information in a matter of seconds than our ancestors might have processed in an entire day.

We are also bombarded with decisions and tasks to complete on a daily basis, from what to eat for lunch to how to respond to your boss's "URGENT" email and what to make of the politically charged articles that appear in your news feed. Your mind is being put to work for long hours every day, and instead of going to sleep when the sun goes down, most of us tend to stay up into the wee hours watching Netflix, staring at more artificial light, and continuing to fill our brains with more and more information in an attempt to relax.

Of course your brain is overloaded. The term for this collective barrage is **technostress**, which quickly leads to serious issues like impaired decision making, poor memory retrieval, a decline in your cognitive function, and elevated stress levels. It also affects your daily performance and learning efficiency. And to escape from it all, most people go look at another screen to distract themselves, which only makes the problem worse!

To get a bit more specific, technostress leads to a mental state called **cognitive overload**, which is defined as "the point where demands on working memory exceed its capacity, which leads to impaired learning and performance." This comes from the cognitive load theory, which suggests that your working memory has limited bandwidth, and you experience negative effects when it is exceeded.

> Your **working memory** is a cognitive system that allows you to temporarily hold and manipulate information in your mind. It is used for tasks like reasoning, comprehension, and learning.

In other words, there's a limit to how much information your brain can efficiently process at a time, and once you exceed this limit, your performance falls off—often drastically. This is why you might feel mentally exhausted at the end of a hard day or hit a wall while working on a complex project, when you feel like you just can't make any more progress. This isn't just a feeling but a well-documented phenomenon, and it's a serious problem not only for your individual wellbeing, but for our society as a whole.

Think about the impact this impairment has on employees' performance in the workplace and how that translates to the global economy, future inventions (which ironically further the progression of technology and increase technostress), and in critical situations such as healthcare or aviation where even a small mistake could be potentially lethal. Your brain is simply not designed to process information at this speed or frequency, nor in this format, yet societal demands continue to mount.

Case in point: I will never forget my first twenty-four-hour call as a junior neurology resident. I had four pagers (which, for the Gen-Zers reading this, were little square objects from the Stone Age that could only transmit or receive a small strip of text such as a phone number or a brief line of text). Each pager corresponded to a list of twenty-five to forty patients that I was responsible for. This would have been difficult enough for a seasoned doctor, but as a junior trainee it was far more than I could safely handle on my own. In fact, being awake for twenty-four hours without sleep is equivalent to the level of impairment of a blood alcohol concentration of 0.10 percent, which is well above the legal limit to drive in most states. Between this and the known detrimental effects of irregular sleep, it still blows my mind that the medical community not only allows but supports this schedule for trainees—it unfortunately tends to be a mindset of "I did it, and so can you."

You may recall from Chapter 2 that despite the 11 million bits of information that your brain receives every second, you can only focus on or process 50 bits at a time. This is held within your working memory, which can only really allow you to focus on one task at a time. (Which, by the way, is why you may have heard the phrase "multitasking is impossible." It's true: your brain is literally wired to reliably perform one task well at a given time.)

Until you have mastered a task and it becomes part of your implicit memory, it takes substantial effort to focus on and learn it. Think about the first time you rode a bicycle or drove a car. At the time, those activities took nearly all your focus and attention. Now you drive to work every day and arrive without thinking about it—probably while sipping a latte, talking on the phone, or listening to a podcast—all while worrying about the to-do list you need to accomplish and navigating your 70,000 other daily thoughts.

So, what can you do about this? While you can't stop technological change or realistically cut technology completely out of your life—neither of which I would recommend even if you could due to its unquestionable potential for a net improvement in your quality of life—you *can* take control of your own routine and create an effective system that works for you.

As we've covered, running your brain is an energy-intensive process. Like a car, you cannot perform at the red line or max RPM indefinitely. The nice thing is that we all intuitively know that. We feel the effects of it and inherently know when it's causing problems.

There are a variety of techniques you can use to combat technostress and cognitive overload, many of which you've likely heard about on social media if your feed looks anything like mine. To start, research shows that maximal learning and work productivity occurs in intervals of about ninety minutes, and after that performance rapidly declines. This is called your **ultradian rhythm**. So, working in ninety-minute sessions with ten-to-fifteen-minute breaks in between is a great way to not only get more done but keep your brain healthy.

Meditation is another intervention that has plenty of evidence behind it. The regular practice of mindfulness has even been associated with a significant increase in telomerase function. **Telomerase** is an enzyme that repairs your telomeres, which are protective caps at the ends of the chromosomes in your DNA. To make a long story short, preserving your telomeres is another key way to slow the aging process (which is why telomere dysfunction is one of the hallmarks of aging we'll discuss in the next chapter). As a side note, how amazing is that? You can literally heal your cells with the power of your mind—not woo-woo, but actual science.

When it comes to cognitive overload, anything that lowers your stress levels, gets you away from screens, and frees up your brain will be helpful. The less you have to keep track of in your head, the better off you'll be. If you're looking for specifics on how to alleviate technostress, we'll cover some basic principles in Chapter 8, and you can even head to TranscendHealthGroup.com/Resources for a downloadable list of interventions including digital detoxes, breathwork, and more.

Small adjustments to the way you use technology in your daily life can also have profound effects on your mental clarity, stress levels, and ultimately, your longevity. Much like cardiovascular disease and neuroinflammation, the effects of technostress compound over time, making it essential to treat this uniquely modern threat with the same gravity as any other health concern.

GOING DEEPER

We've now explored the four primary threats to your longevity: cardiovascular disease, neurodegenerative disease, neuroinflammation, and technostress. While some of this information may feel sobering or even depressing, I hope you've seen the silver lining: nearly all these conditions are preventable, the risk factors are interrelated, and there's substantial evidence on how to lower your risk.

The reality is that, while we may be dealing with significant health problems as a society, we are living in a unique moment in human history. Never before have we understood these mechanisms so thoroughly, and never before have we had such clear evidence about how to manipulate them. Your grandparents and even your parents likely viewed heart disease and dementia as an unavoidable part of growing older. Today, we know better. You have knowledge and resources at your disposal that previous generations could only dream of, placing you in an unprecedented position to take control of your health trajectory.

Better yet, the interventions required to prevent these conditions are surprisingly straightforward and interrelated. Regular exercise, a whole food diet rich in plants, protein, and healthy fats, adequate sleep, and stress management can lower your risk or prevent these problems from occurring in the first place. Each positive choice you make likely affects multiple areas of your body and therefore combats several of these threats at once. I would not look at these as individual threats to be dealt with, but as the likely consequences of a generally unhealthy lifestyle. The more positive lifestyle changes you can make, the less you'll have to worry about any of these.

Now, if you're feeling a bit confused about any of these mechanisms, don't worry. In the next chapter, we're going to explore the hallmarks of aging, where you'll gain a deeper understanding of the cellular and molecular processes underlying them. By the end, the connections between these unique processes, and the interventions to avoid them will become even clearer. This knowledge will empower you to make more informed decisions about your health, knowing exactly why each choice matters in the grand scheme of your longevity journey.

Rather than fearing these conditions or accepting them as inevitable, you can approach them with confidence, armed with the understanding that your daily choices have the power to shape your future health. I, for one, find that incredibly motivating—and I think you will, too.

KEY TAKEAWAYS

1. **Cardiovascular disease, neurodegenerative disease, neuroinflammation, and technostress represent the four biggest threats to your longevity,** and they share common mechanisms and risk factors. Understanding these connections means that addressing one threat often helps prevent others, as well.

2. **Many of these conditions develop silently over decades before symptoms appear,** which is why prevention through lifestyle choices is far more effective than waiting for problems to develop. Traditional Western medicine often fails us by focusing on treating diseases after they occur rather than preventing them in the first place.

3. **Each of these primary threats is largely preventable through consistent lifestyle interventions.** Regular exercise, proper nutrition, adequate sleep, and stress management can dramatically reduce your risk across all four categories, potentially adding decades of healthy life. And while these are the most impactful, there are even more interventions that will be covered in Part 2.

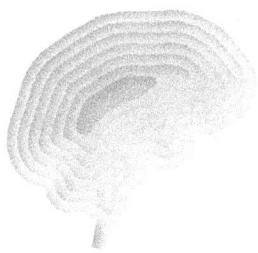

CHAPTER 4
THE HALLMARKS OF AGING

AS AN INPATIENT neurohospitalist, most of my clinical work involves meeting with brand new patients. Therefore, like many doctors, I spend a lot of time reviewing a patient's chart before I walk into their hospital room. This is a critical part of my job because I need to understand how their entire medical history relates to their current symptoms to make the appropriate diagnosis and treatment plan. Usually, I have enough detail to form a relatively narrow differential diagnosis before I walk in the door and in some ways can already envision who a given patient is and what they look like.

That was not the case with Nancy. Not at all.

Nancy's chart indicated that she was a forty-nine-year-old woman with some run-of-the-mill chronic medical issues that had unfortunately led to a minor stroke. Given her relatively young age, I didn't anticipate any significant age-related problems. That's why my first thought upon opening her door was, "Surely, I'm in the wrong room."

There was no way this woman was forty-nine years old. At first glance, I would've sworn the woman in bed was at least eighty. *Not to worry*, I thought. When patients are transported to other departments in the hospital for various diagnostic tests, I often encounter family and friends waiting in their rooms. Surely, this must have been the patient's mother or some older relative waiting for her to return (although that still didn't quite compute given this person was in bed in a hospital gown). As I greeted her, I smiled, introduced myself, and asked her name. She smiled back and confirmed that she was indeed who I had been consulted to see.

How, I thought to myself, could this poor woman appear *so* much older than her actual age? As I heard her story, it all started to make sense. She told me that she suffered from chronic stress for years as a result of her anxiety, which never seemed adequately treated. To cope with this, she had smoked at least two packs of cigarettes a day for the last thirty years. On top of this, she had also experimented with a variety of recreational drugs and alcohol in an attempt to calm her nerves, as well.

When I asked what her sleep was like, she laughed—which induced a brief coughing fit—and with a raspy voice answered, "Oh honey, I wouldn't know what sleep is."

When I asked about her diet, it consisted of almost entirely prepackaged, processed, and fast food. Exercise was a foreign concept. What saddened me most, however, was when I asked about her support system. She teared up and said, "I live alone, I have no friends, and no one loves me."

Trying my best to stifle my emotion, my throat tightened and my eyes watered as I did my best to comfort her. The unfortunate reality for Nancy was that she had done just about everything one ought *not* to do to enjoy a longer life, and sadly most of this was in the form of coping with one problem or another that was entirely treatable. This sequence of events over a period of years had now resulted in very real consequences, and there was no doubt her life would ultimately be shortened as a result. The fact that she had made it until forty-nine without a prior major health event like a heart attack or stroke was almost a miracle in and of itself.

Nancy's story stands in stark contrast to Robert's, the spry 103-year-old man we met in Chapter 1 who went dancing three times a week with his wife and woke up every day with a purpose. When I talk about changes to your lifestyle and their compounding effects over time, this is precisely what's at stake. You will inevitably age (barring any major changes in the future, which we'll discuss in Chapter 10), but the *rate* at which you age is largely up to you. Once you understand the mechanisms at play, you'll see that aging is really just the cumulative effect of multiple interconnected processes, all of which can be substantially modified by lifestyle interventions, for better or worse.

That is the focus of this chapter. Together, we'll look at the twelve hallmarks of aging and the cellular mechanisms behind them. Many of these will relate back to the four primary threats of the last chapter, giving you an even deeper understanding of why those problems occur in the first place and how you can prevent them. By the end of this chapter, you'll be equipped with a breadth of knowledge that should serve you well into your future, because once you understand the mechanisms at play, you'll be able to evaluate new interventions as the science advances, understand how they might impact your health, and make more informed decisions regarding what's best for you.

With that said, before we get into the hallmarks of aging, it would be a good idea to clarify what *aging* actually means.

WHAT IS AGING?

Aging is something we all experience. With the passage of time, we all share the familiar signs of gray hair, wrinkles, and the inevitable slowing of various organ systems. These superficial changes, however, are merely indirect representations of what's actually happening within your body on a cellular level.

Biologically speaking, aging is really just a collection of interconnected cellular mechanisms that gradually change your cells, tissues, and organs over time, and not for the better. As mentioned previously, aging is the single greatest risk factor for neurodegenerative diseases like Alzheimer's and Parkinson's, cardiovascular disease, diabetes, and cancer—because as your cells age, the mechanisms in your body begin to falter, and problems begin to accumulate.

Therefore, slowing your rate of aging at the cellular level is perhaps your best chance to ensure optimal longevity and keep your brain and body performing well so you can do more of what you love for as long as possible. There is, however, an important conceptual distinction to be made with respect to aging. When we talk about birthdays passing by, that is what is referred to as **chronological aging**—a number that is arbitrarily measured on a calendar. Your **biological age,** however, refers to a much more complex series of changes occurring at a molecular level throughout your entire body. While it's true that your chronological age largely correlates with an older biological age, they are not completely interdependent upon one another.

One example of this is a rare condition called Hutchinson-Gilford progeria syndrome. While uncommon and caused by a genetic mutation, this results in dramatically accelerated biological aging with an average life expectancy of just fifteen years of age. If you would like a profound perspective on life from someone who had this condition, look up the TEDx talk by Sam Berns, who was just seventeen at the time he delivered it. It's called "My Philosophy for a Happy Life," and as of this writing, it has over 54 million views on YouTube. Just be sure to bring your tissue box.

Rare genetic exceptions aside, the rate at which you age is largely a result of your daily actions. Which begs the question: Is aging inevitable?

IS AGING INEVITABLE?

As of 2025, the average life expectancy at birth for both sexes globally was 73.5 years, with females living to an average age of 75 years and males living to an average age of 71 years. There's no definitive scientific explanation for the gender gap, though I have my own theory that it has something to do with the "hold my beer" phenomenon that seems more prevalent among males, which when thinking back to stunts in my younger years, certainly holds up.

Since the 1840s, developments in medical technology and public health have added approximately 2.5 years of life per decade, or about three months for every year that we're alive. For reference, the average human life expectancy in 1900 was *just 32 years*, and if the current trend continues, life expectancy by 2050 is estimated to be 78 years.

Furthermore, the majority of current evidence suggests that survival rates decline substantially after age one hundred, and that we experience a sharp physiologic decline and loss of overall functional capacity by age eighty for those who even make it that far. This would appear to suggest there's a natural limit to the human lifespan, and in either case, we accept aging as part of the normal process of life because for as long as humans have existed, this has been an observed phenomenon with which we are all familiar.

But what if aging were optional? Or at least dramatically modifiable? It's difficult to say whether this could ever be feasible in reality, but if we consider other species, this concept does seem biologically plausible. The glass sponge, for example, is believed to live between 10,000 and 15,000 years (yes, *thousand*). Black coral has a known lifespan of over 5,000 years, and there are examples of ancient bristlecone pine trees known to be at least 5,000 years old, which are still going strong. The Greenland shark, which is the longest known living vertebrate in the world, has a lifespan of up to 500 years.

One of my personal favorites is the giant tortoise, which is believed to live up to 250 years and is the oldest known land-dwelling animal. The oldest known giant tortoise as of this writing is a 193-year-old resident of the Seychelles Islands named Jonathan. To put this into perspective, Jonathan has lived through the reign of 40 US presidents and was alive nearly 30 years before the start of the American Civil War.

To state the obvious, there are quite a few differences between a human and a glass sponge, but far less so between us and other vertebrates. That said, we are all carbon-based organisms whose physical bodies are encoded by the same underlying molecular substrate, DNA. In either case, there's tremendous disagreement within the scientific community around whether humans have a natural upper limit or not. Predicting the future of human longevity is difficult for obvious reasons, but one core problem is that our brains are hardwired to think in linear fashion.

There are likely evolutionary reasons for this. (Here it is again! You really should write your ancestors a thank-you card.) Making tools, starting a fire, and hunting prey all require a series of linear planning and step-by-step execution, which your ancestors' brains (and subsequently yours) would naturally follow. Today, we experience most of life unfolding in a linear fashion and we even measure time this way. Technology, however, progresses *exponentially* over time—which is very difficult for us to wrap our heads around given the way we are programmed to think.

THE TECHNOLOGY EXPLOSION

The **Law of Accelerating Returns** states that technological progress tends to increase exponentially over time. This term was originally coined by Ray Kurzweil, a computer scientist, futurist, and inventor. According to this theory, the initial rate of technological progress was so slow that this wouldn't appear to be true, but for those familiar with the idea of compounding returns, we're now starting to see that Kurzweil's theory may in fact hold water.

Technology has continued to progress rapidly over the course of my lifetime, and it doesn't appear to be stopping any time soon. For example, in 2023, ChatGPT passed the MCAT (Medical College Admissions Test) required for admission to medical school. This brutal exam takes a well-trained human over seven hours to get through, including breaks, and months of rigorous preparation (I've done it and I'm glad I don't have to ever again). It also passed all three steps of the United States Medical Licensing Exams (USMLE) required to practice medicine and surpassed a 90 percent accuracy in medical diagnosis, outperforming most physicians on the same tests. And it did all of this almost instantaneously.

As these technologies continue to improve, they are being applied to drug discovery, research, and interventions that may slow, halt, or even reverse aspects of cellular aging that we once thought were inevitable. Given our pattern of linear-thinking and current limited worldview, it's almost impossible to predict what might happen in the next two, five, or ten years—but I think it's safe to say the future of longevity looks incredibly promising, and I am confident there are serious breakthroughs on the horizon. If these come to pass, they will likely have a dramatic effect on the way we age and will probably force me to write another book just to stay up to date.

That said, I don't think waiting around for technology to solve your problems is a strong solution. The reality is that even if there are major breakthroughs, the tried-and-true methods will always work because that is how you are designed. Therefore, you should likely focus on what you can do right now with the knowledge we already have (which is extensive) to give yourself the best chance possible to age well and be in optimal health when the future arrives. For now, this means achieving a basic understanding and addressing the fundamental mechanisms of aging that science has already identified.

These mechanisms, known as the "hallmarks of aging," are the cellular and molecular processes that drive age-related physical and cognitive decline. Understanding them and implementing evidence-based steps to slow their progression is perhaps the best overall strategy we currently have for slowing your own rate of aging. So, let's explore these hallmarks and how you can influence them through your daily choices.

THE HALLMARKS OF AGING

While this can get quite complex and there are likely additional mechanisms we've still yet to discover, current evidence shows that there are twelve main hallmarks of aging that we should all be concerned with. These are processes that are happening in your body right now that will determine how well you'll age in the coming years and decades, and all of them can be heavily influenced through lifestyle choices.

It is crucial to know that most of these hallmarks go largely undetected in your body for long periods before the first symptom ever appears. As we've mentioned, your body is well adapted to buffer cumulative damage while keeping you functioning well, even when things begin to falter at the cellular level. This is why sudden medical events like cancer diagnoses or heart attacks often appear entirely out of the blue, even to people who are seemingly healthy. But the reality is that these hallmarks of aging were silently at work without anyone knowing it.

You will not be able to read through this list and think, *Yes, that one is happening to me,* or, *Nope, I don't have to worry about this one*—and that's kind of the point. Most of these hallmarks are happening to all of us on some level as they are by definition the inevitable result of aging, which is the current price of admission to this thing we call life.

However, you can largely control the rate at which they progress through your chosen lifestyle. For each hallmark, I'll start with a simplified, high-level explanation then dig into the specifics. At the end of each explanation, I will then offer a few interventions for you to consider. If you'd like to skip ahead or you feel yourself getting bogged down in the details here, feel free to peruse the high-level explanations and move on to the next chapter where we'll begin to cover specific interventions in greater detail.

#1: CHRONIC INFLAMMATION

By now, you should have a solid understanding of inflammation, but it's worth revisiting as it's one of the most impactful hallmarks of aging, and one that we will continue to address with many interventions in coming chapters.

Imagine your body's immune system as a security team. When there's a threat like a cut or infection, this team springs into action, neutralizes the danger, heals things up, and then stands down. That's acute inflammation, and it's essential for your survival. Chronic inflammation is what happens when this security team keeps unnecessarily kicking in doors. They remain on high alert indefinitely, which puts *a lot* of unnecessary stress on your body, resulting in collateral damage. Over time, this persistent, low-grade inflammation can damage your cells, tissues, and organs, accelerating aging and increasing disease risk.

You've certainly experienced inflammation before. When you stub your toe, it swells and hurts, and you can feel inflammation in your body in real time. Chronic inflammation, however, can fly under the radar—you don't always notice when it's happening to you. This constant, low-grade inflammatory state can result in what's called **inflammaging** (when inflammation causes accelerated aging, hence the literal combination of "inflammation and aging") which contributes to nearly every age-related disease, from heart disease to dementia.

Specific inflammatory-related diseases include:

- Type 2 diabetes
- Non-alcoholic fatty liver disease
- Cancer
- Autoimmune disease
- Neurodegenerative diseases such as Parkinson's and Alzheimer's
- Cardiovascular diseases such as atherosclerosis and congestive heart failure

One way to think about inflammation is that your body naturally seeks an optimal balance to keep you functioning well—a state called **homeostasis**. So, when you experience negative stressors like a poor diet or physical inactivity, your body is forced to burn additional resources to maintain this balance and keep you alive. This poses a serious opportunity cost as the energy spent fighting these avoidable stressors can't be used in other areas to keep things operating at their full potential, such as repairing your DNA, regulating your metabolism, or keeping your cells younger.

The problem is that far too many aspects of modern life keep your immune system in this state of constant activation. Processed foods, sedentary behavior, chronic stress, poor sleep, and environmental toxins all trigger inflammatory responses that never fully resolve. When your body experiences these negative stressors for long periods of time, it's like putting the aging accelerator pedal to the floor. Your body ends up constantly wasting energy and resources fighting back against an enemy that it will never defeat. Therefore, the best method at your disposal is to not let the enemy enter in the first place! Before we cover these in more detail in the following chapters, here are a few interventions to get you thinking.

Evidence-Based Interventions:
- An anti-inflammatory diet rich in colorful fruits and vegetables, healthy fats (especially omega-3s), and minimize ultra-processed foods
- Regular exercise—even moderate activity—has potent anti-inflammatory effects
- Stress management through practices like meditation, yoga, or time in nature
- Adequate sleep, which helps regulate immune function
- Minimized exposure to environmental toxins when possible

#2: CELLULAR SENESCENCE

Cellular senescence is the accumulation of cells that have stopped dividing but remain metabolically active and secrete pro-inflammatory cytokines which can damage surrounding tissues. (You may recall cytokines from our discussion of traumatic brain injuries in Chapter 3—excess pro-inflammatory cytokines are problematic.)

One way to think about this is as your cells age, they sometimes reach a point where they can no longer divide—which is a normal part of a cell's life cycle—but they don't die, either, which is not normal. These cells enter this so-called senescent state, and are often referred to as "zombie cells," which is an apt description (and quite frankly, kind of gross).

As their name implies, these zombie cells don't just hang out—they're actively harmful, as the excess cytokines they secrete cause inflammation, which is just one of many examples of how these hallmarks are all interrelated. Zombie cells also become resistant to **apoptosis**, which is how other unhealthy cells become marked for destruction when they ultimately wear out. So not only are they actively harmful, but your body is unable to detect them. That means senescent cells often persist for extended periods of time, which is not ideal.

So, what causes these zombie cells? Senescence is mostly thought to be triggered by DNA damage including telomere dysfunction, oxidative stress, and activation of **oncogenes**, which are genes that cause cancer. To grossly oversimplify this, when your DNA becomes damaged, it can ultimately be misread, which creates problems with the way your cells manufacture proteins. This can eventually lead to the cell becoming senescent.

Due to the inflammation they cause, senescent cells contribute to a wide variety of age-related diseases, including most of the ones we've mentioned thus far.

Evidence-Based Interventions:
- Senolytic compounds can help clear senescent cells. These include:
    - Quercetin (onions, apple, berries)
    - Fisetin (strawberries)
    - Curcumin (turmeric)
    - Resveratrol (in supplement form—not red wine)

#3: LOSS OF PROTEOSTASIS

Proteins are the fundamental building blocks of life. You, me, and every carbon-based organism on the planet are primarily made of protein (by dry weight anyway, meaning without the water), from our organs down to the microscopic components within each cell.

When we zoom in to a single cell, we find an intricate factory-like system with various **organelles** (specialized structures) that each serve unique functions. If you took biology in high school, you probably covered most of the big ones, like **ribosomes** (which manufacture proteins), **lysosomes** (which break down waste materials), and **mitochondria** (which generate energy, as previously discussed), to name a few. All these organelles must work in harmony, which involve proteins constantly being created, folded, transported, and degraded in a delicate balance.

That delicate balance is called proteostasis. Loss of proteostasis therefore occurs when the balance is disrupted. This can happen in several ways:

- Problems with protein production, where proteins aren't synthesized correctly

- Issues with protein folding, where proteins don't achieve their proper three-dimensional structure
- Failures in protein degradation, where damaged or unnecessary proteins aren't properly removed

When proteostasis is lost, misfolded or damaged proteins can accumulate within cells, causing problems. This is exactly what happens in Parkinson's disease, where alpha-synuclein builds up inside neurons, which interferes with normal neuronal function, eventually triggering cell death.

Imagine this type of thing happening in varying degrees of severity across the trillions of cells throughout your body. In your brain, it can lead to neurodegenerative disease, but across your body, it can cause an endless array of problems, including many of the chronic diseases we've covered so far. This is why loss of proteostasis is such a critical hallmark of aging and why you've already heard the phrase many times leading up to this chapter. It affects virtually every aspect of your cellular function.

Your body has multiple quality control systems designed to help you maintain proteostasis, but as you age, they become less efficient—partly due to some of the other hallmarks we'll discuss throughout this chapter. However, certain lifestyle interventions can help you maintain and even enhance these protective mechanisms.

Evidence-Based Interventions:
- Regular exercise, which stimulates autophagy and enhances cellular cleanup processes
- Calorie restriction or intermittent fasting, which has been shown to improve protein quality control
- Adequate protein intake

- Consumption of foods rich in polyphenols like green tea, berries, and olive oil
- Sufficient sleep, which is when much of the cellular cleanup occurs
- Stress management, as chronic stress can impair proteostasis
- Sauna bathing, as heat shock proteins play a key role in proteostasis

#4: DEREGULATED NUTRIENT SENSING

Your body has an incredibly sophisticated system for absorbing and distributing nutrients. When you eat food, the macronutrients—proteins, carbs, and fats—enter this system and are ultimately transported to various locations throughout your body. Nutrients pass from your mouth through your stomach, are mostly absorbed into your body by your intestines, then pass through the liver where some are stored; however, the vast majority are delivered to the rest of the organs in your body like your muscles or your brain. These nutrients essentially become the building blocks of your body—which is why the phrase "you are what you eat" is incredibly accurate. You are literally made up of the molecules you ingest, just in a slightly different final form—an amino acid from a ribeye steak becoming part of your right bicep, for example.

When this system works properly, every calorie has a specific job and destination. Your body has checkpoints, receptors, and pathways that direct nutrients where they need to go. It's an intricate symphony of chemical messengers ensuring that energy is properly distributed, stored, and utilized.

But as we age or make less-than-ideal lifestyle choices, this finely tuned system begins to falter. Essentially, your body starts putting things where they don't belong. The result is an impaired metabolism and disrupted energy balance. This disruption can manifest in several ways, including:

- Improper storage of nutrients
- Failure to build muscle efficiently
- Excess fat, particularly visceral fat around your organs, which can trigger more inflammation
- Increased fasting blood sugar and insulin resistance

Essentially, when the various nutrient-sensing systems in your body do not receive the proper amount of energy (too little or too much) over time problems arise. In our modern world, the predominant issue most people experience is excess energy from being over-nourished.

When you consume more calories than you need, a pathway called **mTOR** becomes over-activated—the pathway responsible for growth and energy storage. While mTOR is absolutely necessary for building and repairing parts of your body, its chronic over-activation creates a cascade of problems: increased inflammation, higher blood pressure, greater insulin resistance, elevated cholesterol...and ultimately increases your risk for diabetes, heart attacks, strokes, Alzheimer's, and many other conditions. As you can imagine, this has also been associated with a decreased lifespan.

We'll cover mTOR in greater depth in Chapter 6, so all you really need to know now is that consuming excess calories for long periods of time keeps this pathway in a perpetual "on" state, which isn't great for most people.

The causes of deregulated nutrient sensing are multifaceted and, once again, interconnected with other processes. Poor diet and physical inactivity are the primary culprits, but aging itself plays a role as your metabolic pathways naturally slow down and become less efficient over time. Other contributing factors include oxidative stress, which can damage your cells through free radical formation, and chronic inflammation, which also disrupts normal metabolic signaling.

Evidence-Based Interventions:
- Mindfulness of overall calories in and calories out—what you eat vs. what you burn
- Time-restricted eating or intermittent fasting, which can help reset nutrient sensing pathways
- Regular exercise, particularly a combination of resistance training and cardiovascular activity
- Adequate protein intake while avoiding excess calorie consumption
- Sufficient micronutrients, particularly those that support metabolic health, like magnesium and B vitamins
- Quality sleep, which plays a crucial role in metabolic regulation
- Minimized consumption of ultra-processed foods that can disrupt metabolic signaling

#5: MITOCHONDRIAL DYSFUNCTION

Your mitochondria are the microscopic power plants within your cells that generate the majority of your body's energy currency, called adenosine triphosphate (ATP).

To put into perspective how important this process is, cyanide—the classic poison you've probably seen in movies—works by blocking one of the enzymes within the electron transport chain in the mitochondria (cytochrome c oxidase, for those interested). This instantaneously halts ATP production throughout the entire body and can literally kill you within minutes. So, please leave this to the James Bond villains and don't try experimenting with cyanide at home. Jokes aside, this illustrates the importance of your mitochondria and why it's in your best interest to keep them functioning optimally.

If your mitochondria were to stop working entirely, you'd die in seconds, but when their function is simply impaired, the symptoms are far more subtle. Mitochondrial dysfunction can result in low energy levels within your cells and an increase in **reactive oxygen species,** both of which damage adjacent structures and can contribute to premature aging. If your mitochondria are severely impaired, this can also trigger apoptosis, or programmed cell death.

> **Reactive oxygen species** are unstable oxygen molecules that can create chemical reactions in the body which cause damage. Without going too deep into the chemistry, these oxygen molecules don't have the proper pairs and number of electrons in their orbit. **Antioxidants** can bind and stabilize reactive oxygen species, mitigating their damage—which is why you often hear about them in relation to longevity.

Mitochondrial dysfunction can occur for various reasons: environmental stressors, mutations in your mitochondrial DNA, chronic disease, or cellular senescence. The effects can be wide-ranging, impacting everything from your heart to your brain.

For instance, metabolic diseases like type 2 diabetes strongly correlate with mitochondrial dysfunction. Cardiovascular conditions, including coronary artery disease and heart failure, are linked to damage in heart muscle cells and blood vessels due to impaired mitochondrial function. Even cancer can result from dysfunction in the Krebs cycle, the main pathway through which your body produces ATP. This disruption can lead to mitochondrial DNA mutations and increased formation of tumor cells.

Evidence-Based Interventions:
- Regular exercise
- Consuming antioxidant-rich foods
- A proper nutrition plan
- Creatine monohydrate supplementation

#6: DISABLED MITOPHAGY

When we discussed neurodegenerative disease in Chapter 3, we touched on a process called autophagy (which literally means "self-eating"). This is the process your cells use to recycle damaged components. We also briefly touched on mitophagy, a similar process that targets the mitochondria within your cells. There are hundreds to thousands of mitochondria within each of your cells, and they will naturally incur damage over time. When this reaches the point of no return, so to speak, mitophagy is the process by which your cells chew them up and recycle them.

This is essentially the "check" for mitochondrial dysfunction, our previous hallmark. When this mechanism is functioning properly, your cells will chew up and recycle any dysfunctional mitochondria—which is great! But when it isn't, damaged and dysfunctional mitochondria accumulate, which leads to the same problems as previously discussed (cellular dysfunction, oxidative stress, and eventually the death of the cell through apoptosis), or perhaps worse: cellular senescence.

Going back to our powerhouse analogy and thinking of your mitochondria as your cellular engines, the process of mitophagy is like having a mechanic. When things go wrong with your engine (mitochondrial dysfunction) you call your mechanic to fix it. It's a great system, until one day when your mechanic seems to be mysteriously sick half the time you call him (disabled mitophagy). Now your poorly maintained engine starts having even more problems and your car (body) doesn't run well. Side note: keep up with your oil changes!

In your brain in particular, impaired mitophagy can also result in premature neuronal cell death, contributing to the development of neurodegenerative diseases. Similarly, in other organ systems it can also lead to metabolic disorders, cardiovascular disease, and even cancer.

The interventions for disabled mitophagy are essentially the same as those for mitochondrial dysfunction.

#7: STEM CELL EXHAUSTION

Stem cells are your body's repair and regeneration specialists. And before we go too deep, it's worth clarifying a common misconception, which is that *you naturally have stem cells within your body right now—* they're not something you need to obtain from an external source.

Stem cells are essentially younger versions of your cells that don't have a specialization quite yet. They're cells without a specific job, waiting for instructions on what to become. In general, you have more stem cells when you're younger, and they have a greater capacity to differentiate into various tissues as needed such as eye cells, skin cells, and muscle cells.

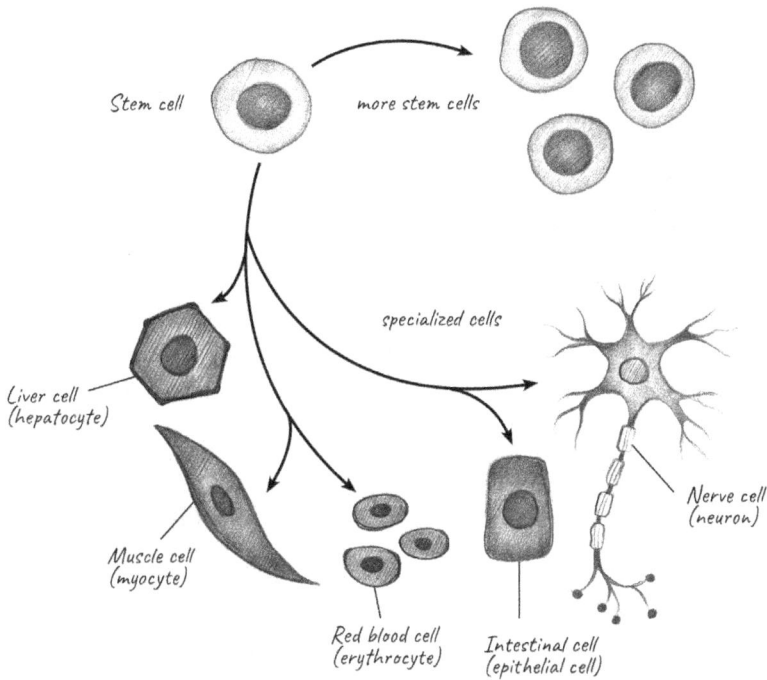

DIAGRAM 8: *Different types of stem cells*

There are also different types of stem cells along a spectrum of specialization. Take blood cells as an example. At the top of the development chart is what's called a **multipotent hematopoietic stem cell** (say that five times fast). This single cell type can eventually become any of the circulating immunologic cells in your body—natural killer cells, lymphocytes, neutrophils, and many others. Before these stem cells decide what they're going to be, they exist in a common, undeveloped state. Depending on where they end up or what signals they receive, they can turn into any number of specialized cells.

We all have resident stem cells living in our tissues. These cells help with both repair and routine maintenance by dividing, reproducing, and generating new copies of themselves that then develop into specialized tissue cells. This process is tissue-specific. Muscle and brain tissue, for example, don't turn over very often, while skin and intestinal cells regenerate constantly. This also explains why a sore in your mouth heals within a day or two, while a torn muscle or tendon can take weeks or months to heal properly. The rate of stem cell activity and tissue regeneration varies dramatically throughout the body.

As we age or experience chronic health problems, our stem cells can become exhausted. Chronic stress, underlying disease, and persistent inflammation can further accelerate that process, causing stem cells to enter a senescent state where they no longer proliferate effectively. This exhaustion affects your ability to repair injuries, but more importantly, it can hinder the day-to-day maintenance of our organs.

For example, some of your liver cells naturally incur damage and die as part of their normal life cycle. Your local stem cells help turn those over and generate new liver cells to maintain the organ's overall function. When your stem cells become exhausted, however, your liver can no longer work as well, which it turns out is crucial to your survival.

As a side note, while stem cell therapy (injecting foreign donor stem cells into your body or harvesting and injecting your own) shows promise for certain applications, it's important to understand what's currently supported by evidence. Bone marrow transplants are perhaps the most established stem cell treatment, used primarily for blood cancers with life-saving results. There's also emerging research on stem cell applications for cartilage regeneration, wound healing, and joint repair. The idea is that injecting stem cells into damaged areas might speed up repair processes that would normally take much longer. Cartilage and joint tissues, which typically heal very slowly, are particular targets for this research.

While there are many potential future applications (enhanced recovery from TBIs, improving spinal cord injuries, and nerve regrowth, to name a few), much of the current stem cell therapy landscape exists outside FDA approval. Many treatments are available in countries outside the US, but as of this writing, the data on their effectiveness for extending human lifespan is still fairly limited.

The moral of the story is that injecting stem cells will likely not be a defining factor in your longevity journey—at least for now. In addition to their limited use-cases, they're also prohibitively expensive for many. The truth is that there are many basic, free lifestyle changes with far more robust evidence for improving your longevity outcomes. My preference would be to focus on those fundamentals, which we know have a massive impact, before turning to more costly and experimental interventions like stem cell therapy.

Evidence-Based Interventions:
- Regular physical activity, which appears to maintain stem cell populations in multiple tissues
- Proper nutrition, as stem cells are sensitive to nutrient availability
- Management of chronic inflammation, which can damage stem cell reservoirs
- Adequate sleep, which supports stem cell proliferation
- Time-restricted eating or intermittent fasting, which may help preserve stem cell function

#8: GENOMIC INSTABILITY

Genomic instability refers to the accumulation of DNA damage over time, which leads to DNA mutations and chromosomal abnormalities. While this might sound surprising, your DNA is actually breaking and being repaired constantly, during every minute of every day.

This is a normal part of living. Fortunately, your body has specialized enzymes that faithfully repair your DNA, maintaining your genomic stability under normal conditions.

> A **DNA mutation** is a permanent change in the sequence of your DNA, which can occur spontaneously or be induced by environmental factors. **Chromosomal abnormalities** are epigenetic conditions that result in potential misreading and/or destabilization of the genome.

Before we get into the more scientific details, here's a simple analogy to explain how this works. Think of your DNA as an enormous library containing thousands of instruction books that tell your cells exactly how to function. Every day, this library experiences wear and tear. Some books get damaged from harmful sunlight (UV radiation), others from coffee spills (environmental toxins), and some simply deteriorate with repeated use.

Fortunately, your body employs a team of dedicated librarians (DNA repair enzymes) who constantly patrol the shelves, finding and repairing damaged books. When you're young, this system works remarkably well—there are lots of librarians, they're very good at replacing missing information, and they're extremely thorough. But as you age, the rate of damage increases while your team of librarians decreases both in number and efficiency. This leads to genomic instability—a gradual accumulation of errors in your DNA that aren't being properly repaired.

The problems begin when you experience increased environmental stressors that cause excessive damage to your DNA, overwhelming these repair mechanisms. When you're overexposed to things like UV light, cigarette smoke, environmental pollutants, or even certain processed foods, your body's repair capacity can be exceeded. This can result in more damage to your DNA than your repair machinery can handle, which can lead to genomic instability and eventually mutations. These mutations can cause loss of proteostasis by way of improper gene expression, contributing to premature aging, autoimmune diseases, and even cancer.

For example, there's a rare genetic condition called xeroderma pigmentosum, where people lack a family of enzymes that repair DNA breaks caused by UV light. As a result, these individuals develop severe sunburns, excess freckles, and cataracts after normal sun exposure that would have virtually no noticeable effect on a person without these uncommon genetic mutations. Unfortunately, people with this condition will almost inevitably develop skin cancer, which demonstrates what can happen when these critical cellular mechanisms don't work properly, although this is an extreme example.

Gene expression is the process by which the information encoded in your DNA is used to direct the assembly of a protein molecule.

Your risk of genomic instability increases with age as your repair mechanisms become less efficient and environmental damage accumulates as your cells age. Other factors that can contribute to genomic instability include chronic inflammation, oxidative stress, and certain nutritional deficiencies.

Evidence-Based Interventions:
- Minimized exposure to known DNA-damaging agents like UV radiation, tobacco smoke, and environmental toxins

- Antioxidant-rich foods to combat oxidative stress
- Adequate intake of nutrients involved in DNA repair, including folate, zinc, and vitamins C, D, and E
- Regular exercise, which has been shown to upregulate DNA repair mechanisms
- Proper sleep habits, as sleep deprivation can impair DNA repair

#9: EPIGENETIC ALTERATIONS

Your **epigenome** is the collection of chemical compounds that sit around your DNA and control how your genes are expressed.

Your DNA is arranged as a double helix molecule wrapped tightly on itself, folded into loops called chromatin, and packaged with proteins called histones. When your cells need to read a segment of DNA, like when creating a new cell, this packaging must be partly unraveled. After this happens, your cell can read your DNA and convert it into RNA, which is then used as a template to make the appropriate protein for whatever cellular component is needed. The set of mechanisms responsible for all that packaging, unpackaging, and reading is your epigenome. Epigenetic alterations refer to changes in that process.

If we continue with our library analogy, genomic instability is like damage to the books themselves, while epigenetic alterations affect how the books are organized, accessed, and read. Your epigenome works through several key mechanisms which aren't terribly important to know about, but I'll add them here for the more scientifically inclined readers:

- **DNA methylation:** Adding methyl groups to DNA, which can silence gene expression

- **Histone modification:** Affecting how chromatin is packaged
- **Regulation by non-coding RNAs:** Controlling which genes are expressed

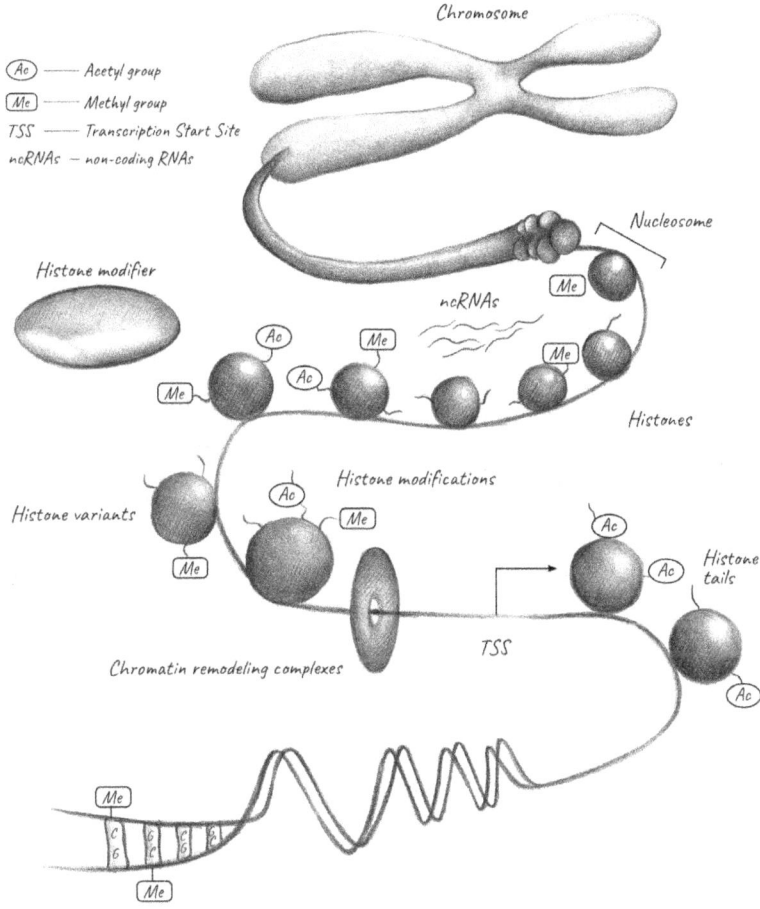

DIAGRAM 9: *DNA (double helix) and the Epigenome*

These processes determine which genes are turned "on" or "off" at any given time, which is crucial for proper cell function. As we age, our epigenetic patterns change, often resulting in improper gene expression, which can contribute to premature aging, autoimmune disease, and cancer.

Interestingly, there's a host of research that has come to light in recent years about the importance of the epigenome regulating your gene expression with regard to longevity. In fact, perhaps one of the easiest and increasingly reliable ways you can test your rate of biological aging is through an epigenetic test that measures your pattern of DNA methylation, which changes over time and demonstrates distinct patterns as we age.

By sending in a cheek swab, a laboratory can compare your pattern of DNA methylation with data sets of older and younger individuals to generate your so-called biological age, an estimated number reflecting your biological rate of aging. If you're sixty years old but your methylation pattern looks similar to what a thirty-year-old's might, then the inference is that you are aging at a slower rate. The goal, therefore, is to have your estimated biological age remain lower than your chronological age.

For instance, I have tested mine on several occasions and received biological age scores between twenty-nine and thirty-three when my chronological age was thirty-six. There are people who obsess over numbers like these, which I'm not quite sure is worth your time yet due to the nascency of such tests. Do I think they represent a perfectly accurate biological age or rate of aging? No. Do I think they're a decent gauge? I think that's likely. I think we'll also likely continue to see improved measurements in the near future that are already being developed, so stay tuned.

Evidence-Based Interventions:
- Regular exercise
- Proper nutrition, and, in particular, receiving adequate micronutrients
- Adequate sleep
- Avoid smoking, alcohol, toxin exposure, environmental pollutants
- Avoiding stress

#10: TELOMERE ATTRITION

Telomere attrition refers to the progressive shortening of your telomeres, which are those protective "end caps" on your chromosomes mentioned previously. You could think of telomeres like the plastic tips on shoelaces—they prevent the ends of your chromosomes from fraying or sticking together, which would damage your DNA, which contains all the genetic information that makes you *you*.

Every time your cells divide, however, your telomeres get a little shorter. This shortening process was once thought to be the primary driver of aging, with researchers in the early 2010s focusing heavily on telomeres as a potential key to extending lifespan. While we now know aging is far more complex, telomere attrition does remain a significant hallmark of the aging process.

As telomeres shorten beyond a critical length, they can no longer protect the ends of your chromosomes effectively. This can lead to genomic instability—therefore, many of the same problems we've just outlined thereby resulting in a gradual decline in cellular function as we age. And while telomere attrition is considered a normal part of aging much like gray hair and wrinkles, the rate at which this occurs can be influenced by a variety of lifestyle factors. Research has shown that certain interventions can help maintain telomere length or slow the rate of shortening.

Evidence-Based Interventions:
- Regular exercise, particularly aerobic activities
- Mediterranean diet rich in omega-3 fatty acids, antioxidants, and fiber
- Intermittent fasting, which has been associated with an *increase* in telomere length in some studies
- Adequate sleep, which supports cellular repair mechanisms
- Stress management, as chronic stress accelerates telomere shortening
- Avoiding tobacco and excessive alcohol consumption
- Maintaining a healthy weight

#11: ALTERED INTERCELLULAR COMMUNICATION

Altered intercellular communication is just as it sounds. Your cells are constantly exchanging information to coordinate the complex functions that keep you alive and healthy. This communication happens through various signaling molecules, which largely include cytokines—the previously mentioned proteins that your cells use to "talk" to each other.

Under normal conditions, cytokines are essential messengers that help regulate immune responses, cell growth, and many other critical functions. Cell one sends a signal to cell two, which is essentially a message telling the second cell to perform a specific function.

This back-and-forth communication creates the coordinated activity necessary to maintain your body's proper function. Without intercellular communication, we wouldn't last very long.

Like many of these systems in our body, however, this communication network can break down as we age. If there's too much communication, too little, or the wrong kind of communication, that can cause problems. One major issue is chronic inflammation, which can lead to an overabundance of those previously mentioned pro-inflammatory cytokines. You could think of this like a room full of people who go from speaking at a normal volume, in an organized fashion, to everyone just yelling at each other. The former is productive, the latter is not and can lead to problems.

As an extreme example, this can rarely escalate to what's called a **cytokine storm**, which is a massive, uncontrolled release of inflammatory cytokines that can be life-threatening, causing rapid drops in blood pressure, multiorgan failure, and even cardiac arrest. While this is another dramatic illustration, it demonstrates how critical proper intercellular communication is to your survival.

The interconnected nature of these communication networks means that disruptions can cascade throughout the body, affecting hormone signaling, immune function, neurological processes, and more. This is why altered intercellular communication is considered a fundamental hallmark of aging—when cells can't communicate effectively, our bodies simply cannot function as they should.

Evidence-Based Interventions:
- Anti-inflammatory diet rich in omega-3 fatty acids, antioxidants, and polyphenols
- Regular exercise, which helps regulate inflammatory cytokine levels

- Adequate sleep, which is essential for proper immune signaling
- Stress management techniques, as chronic stress disrupts normal cellular communication
- Maintaining social connections, which surprisingly has been shown to influence cellular signaling pathways
- Time in nature, which can help normalize various biological signaling pathways

#12: DYSBIOSIS

Dysbiosis refers to an imbalance of the different types of microscopic organisms living in your body—too many of certain types and not enough of others—causing them to work improperly or even against you. This hallmark primarily concerns your gut microbiome, which you're probably familiar with. However, it's worth noting that microorganisms exist throughout your digestive tract, in your mouth, and in any area that interfaces with the outside world. (By the way, your *entire digestive tract* interfaces with the outside world—it is essentially an open tube from start to end.)

The number of bacterial cells in your body is thought to roughly equal your total number of human cells, and they are an important part of how you function (although as we will see, without them it's tough to be your best *you*).

Your gut microbiome is particularly significant and is an important component of what's now called the gut-brain axis, the connection between your gut and brain that we discussed briefly in relation to Parkinson's. The bacteria in your gut produce compounds called postbiotics, including short-chain fatty acids, proteins, and vitamins—all of which help regulate numerous aspects of your health. Remarkably, it is estimated that 90–95 percent of your body's serotonin—a neurotransmitter we typically associate with brain function—is actually manufactured in your gut by these bacteria. They also produce dopamine, GABA, acetylcholine, and other neurotransmitters essential for optimal brain health. For context, GABA is the main inhibitory neurotransmitter in your body and acetylcholine is imperative for movement, nerve-to-nerve signaling, and memory.

The influence of your gut microbiome extends far beyond digestion. Emerging research suggests these bacteria can even influence your behavior, and particularly your eating habits. Scientists have identified a "gut-driven hunger signal" distinct from the traditional brain-regulated hunger mechanisms. In essence, your gut bacteria can communicate when and what they want you to eat, which is a pretty incredible insight into the complex relationship between microorganisms and human behavior. Does this mean bacteria are controlling your body? In a way, I suppose it does. I'll leave it to you to decide whether that is fascinating or terrifying.

Beyond influencing your hunger, your microbiome helps regulate your immune function, protects against cancer, sends signals to your bones and muscles to support muscle building, and helps maintain your brain health. As we age, this delicate balance can become disrupted, leading to dysbiosis.

Several factors can throw this population out of balance. Antibiotics, while necessary for treating certain bacterial infections, can wipe out beneficial bacteria alongside the harmful ones (which is why probiotics are often recommended following antibiotic treatment). Poor dietary choices over time—such as consuming excess processed foods while neglecting fiber-rich vegetables and fruits—can also alter your microbial landscape, increasing inflammatory-promoting bacteria while reducing beneficial species. This increased gut inflammation can then contribute to systemic inflammation, further accelerating your cellular aging.

> **Evidence-Based Interventions:**
> - A diverse, fiber-rich diet with plenty of fruits, vegetables, and fermented foods
> - Limited use of unnecessary antibiotics (when antibiotics are needed, consider probiotic supplementation afterward)
> - Minimal consumption of ultra-processed foods and artificial sweeteners
> - Regular physical activity, which promotes microbial diversity
> - Adequate sleep and stress management, as both can affect gut microbial composition
> - Limited use of antimicrobial products like certain mouthwashes, which can disrupt beneficial oral bacteria that eventually contribute to gut health

FROM MECHANISMS TO INTERVENTIONS

With this last hallmark of aging, we're now closing out the "mechanisms" portion of this book and moving into some of the interventions to consider. When we move beyond the specific complexities, there's one clear commonality here. From cardiovascular disease to altered intercellular communication, and neurodegenerative disease to mitochondrial dysfunction, nearly all the mechanisms we've discussed so far are interrelated in some way. Your body is a complex symphony of highly sophisticated systems that work together on a cellular level to orchestrate your life.

While those systems might seem complicated, there are two overarching lessons I'd like you to take away from this, if nothing else. The first is that the solutions to maintain these systems are inherently simple. Maintaining consistent exercise, achieving quality sleep, consuming a diet of mostly whole and unprocessed foods, and effectively managing your stress throughout your life are enough to ward off or at least dramatically lower your risk of developing many of these problems. Supplements, medications, and other techniques like hormetic stressors can be helpful and should not be discounted, but the biggest levers you have by far are the four mentioned above.

The second overarching lesson is that because these systems are so interrelated, a positive change in one area cascades into many positive changes in other areas. For example, when you engage in regular physical activity, you're not just lowering your risk of cardiovascular disease—you're also enhancing your mitochondrial function, reducing inflammation, preserving your telomere length, and supporting proteostasis—all of which lower your risk of developing other problems.

Personally, I find this motivating, and I hope you do, too. For it means that one small, sustainable change to your lifestyle can, and often does, create interrelated changes within your body with an outsize return for your effort. Little things make a big difference, and those small changes can be negative or positive, as we saw with the contrast between Robert and Nancy.

Robert didn't live a longer life because he understood the hallmarks of aging, but because he had a clear purpose that naturally helped inform his daily choices. Therefore, I would urge you to not get bogged down on the individual hallmarks. It isn't right to think of these as individual systems to be optimized or fixed like parts of a car. Rather, they're the interrelated effects of aging, all of which can be slowed or prevented by living a largely healthy lifestyle. And that, as we know, starts with getting crystal clear on your why.

As we move into Part 2 of this book, we'll be shifting gears from the mechanisms of aging and disease to the interventions to slow down or stop them. I'm sure this is the part you've been waiting for, where we use your new scientific foundation to create practical actions for you to consider integrating into your life. The upcoming chapters will provide a number of evidence-based strategies that have been shown to address the primary threats and hallmarks of aging. We'll be focusing on six key areas: exercise, nutrition, sleep, stress management, supplements, and technology. Each of these elements represent an opportunity for you to take control of how your body ages and in turn maximize both your healthspan and your lifespan.

In each section, we'll start by covering some of the basic science, including why these interventions might help you in your quest for increased longevity and improved performance. Just to be clear, I will not be providing you with a list of step-by-step tactics to implement in your life. I will merely be providing you an overview of what the evidence says—a list of evidence-based interventions that you can then choose whether or not to implement or not in your life if you feel they are aligned with your goals. Thanks to your new knowledge, you should be well-equipped to navigate these decisions.

Throughout the upcoming chapters, I encourage you to keep your why at the front of your mind. Your why serves as both a powerful motivator and a practical filter to help you determine which interventions make the most sense for your unique situation and goals. When you connect these strategies to your deeper purpose, they become more than just health practices—they become meaningful steps toward fulfilling your legacy.

Onward to Part 2 and our first intervention: exercise.

KEY TAKEAWAYS

1. **Cellular aging is the primary driver of age-related disease.** The twelve hallmarks of aging represent interconnected cellular mechanisms that collectively determine how quickly your body ages. Understanding these processes reveals why most age-related diseases are not inevitable, but rather the result of accelerated cellular aging.

2. **These hallmarks are deeply interconnected, creating cascading effects throughout your body.** Positive changes in one area often lead to improvements in others, while negative changes can trigger widespread deterioration. This explains why consistent healthy behaviors can have outsized benefits for longevity—they simultaneously address multiple hallmarks of aging through various pathways, creating compound effects that slow cellular aging across all systems.

3. **Your rate of biological aging is largely within your control.** While chronological aging is inevitable, your biological aging can be significantly modified through lifestyle choices. The interventions we'll discuss in the next chapters can effectively target these hallmarks, potentially adding years or even decades of healthy life by maintaining cellular function and slowing the aging process at its most fundamental level.

PART 2

THE INTERVENTIONS

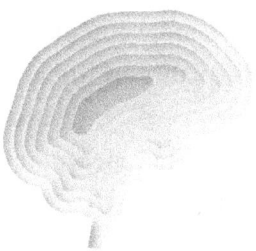

CHAPTER 5
EXERCISE

WHILE I'VE SEEN the transformative power of exercise in my own life and in many of my patients' countless times, there's one recent memory that stands out. A few months ago, I had dinner with my grandfather's former medical partner, Dr. Jim Murphy. At eighty-eight years old, Jim walks with the gait of a thirty-year-old and is sharp as a tack. During our time together, he shared his fascination over the biology textbook he was currently reading. He went on to explain his thoughts on some of the finer points in the text, and frankly, I was having a hard time keeping up with him.

Like I've done with so many of my patients, I asked Jim what his secret was. How had he remained so sharp and physically fit over the years? His answer surprised me. He told me that about a year beforehand, he had actually noticed himself getting weaker, particularly in his legs. He was having trouble getting out of a chair and had to use his arms to push himself up, which was new for him. Given his medical background, he recognized what a serious problem this was—he was at risk of falling, his balance was compromised, and he was becoming increasingly frail.

But instead of accepting this as inevitable, Jim decided to take action. He understood the importance of his physical health and that he would need to be more intentional with his habits if he wanted to maintain his quality of life as he aged. While he was walking several times per week, he wasn't doing any dedicated strength training. So, he started incorporating resistance training into his routine, focusing particularly on leg presses, and within just a few months, experienced a very real transformation.

He'd built noticeable muscle mass in his quadriceps and glutes, which are the muscles that help you resist gravity. As a result, his strength and balance improved dramatically. He mentioned that he had more energy, he felt sharper, and he was getting more done every day. This all happened between the ages of *eighty-seven and eighty-eight*. Jim is the poster child for "it's never too late to start."

THE MAGIC PILL

What if I told you there was a pill that could reduce your risk of dying from any cause by up to 40 percent, cut your risk of heart attack and stroke by nearly 38 percent, and lower your chance of developing dementia by almost 40 percent? One that would improve your mood, sleep quality, and energy levels, while enhancing your cognitive performance and mental clarity? And one that would almost certainly allow you to live a longer, healthier, more vibrant life?

Assuming this pill was safe with minimal side effects, would you take it?

Of course you would. Anyone would. The pharmaceutical company that created such a miracle drug would become the most valuable corporation on Earth overnight.

Here's the thing: this *"pill" already exists. Only it's not a medication—it's exercise.*

If I had to pick one intervention that has the single largest known impact on your brain health and your longevity, it is without a doubt exercise. The benefits are nearly endless. In Part 1, I feared annoying you by listing it out so many times, but it's true that exercise can substantially lower your risk of developing almost all the diseases, conditions, and hallmarks of aging that we've discussed up to this point. Study after study has proven that exercise *is* the magic longevity pill.

The problem is that, unlike a pill you can swallow in seconds, exercise requires your time and effort, which can create resistance. This is part of why it can initially be so difficult to start and maintain a consistent exercise routine. You know what to do, but don't do it because you don't want to sacrifice your valuable time and effort. Or, perhaps, you're already self-conscious about your appearance or lack of knowledge on the subject.

Well, I'm here to tell you that if you want to maximize your time on this earth *and make everything in your life easier*, exercise is the best-known way to do it. It is truly non-negotiable. Exercise is like compound interest for your life. The initial time and energy you invest into exercise upfront will give you far more of both over the course of your life, not to mention all the other things you'll be able to accomplish and enjoy with those resources. It really is that simple, and the best part is it doesn't have to be hard.

In this chapter, our first of the interventions, we're going to cover why exercise is so valuable and how to think about exercise in the context of your life. As you'll see, this does not need to be complicated. You don't need a gym membership, you don't have to become a powerlifter, and you can maintain a consistent routine with minimal time invested. The big lesson I'd like you to take away from this is that *anything is better than nothing*. No matter where you are in your health journey, incorporating any amount of movement into your daily life is good for your long-term health.

The key, as you already know, is making small incremental changes and maintaining consistency over time. The best way to do that, as you also know, is to think back to your purpose—your why—we discussed in Chapter 1. Whether your legacy involves being present for your family, building something meaningful, or making a positive impact on your community, exercise amplifies your ability to fulfill that purpose in endless ways. By maintaining your physical health and cognitive function through regular movement, you're extending not just how long you live, but how long you *live well*. That directly translates into more time and ability to accomplish the things that matter most to you and being able to enjoy them along the way.

Regular exercise will provide you with more energy to meaningfully engage with your loved ones, complete difficult projects, and pursue your passions. You'll think more clearly, solve problems more effectively, and maintain your mental sharpness for far longer.

Being physically fit is also something you'll see value in on a daily basis. Tasks that leave others winded might barely register for you. You'll recover more quickly from illnesses. You'll be able to get more done each day. You'll sleep more soundly. Your mood will be more stable and positive. Even your confidence will grow, thanks to the underlying knowledge that your body is capable of handling most anything that might come your way. All these benefits compound over time, creating a positive feedback loop that improves nearly every aspect of your life.

I can tell you, anecdotally, that I have experienced all these benefits myself for years. But you don't need to take my word for it, just look at the data. According to a 2022 study examining over 100,000 adults, just ten to twenty minutes of vigorous physical activity per day lowered all-cause mortality by 19 percent. Increasing that to forty to sixty minutes per day reduced all-cause mortality by up to 31 percent and cardiovascular disease mortality by up to 38 percent.

A 2022 study in the *Journal of the American Medical Association* looking at over 122,000 people found that those with low cardiorespiratory fitness had a *500 percent increase in mortality risk* compared to the top elite performers. Five. Hundred. Percent! Implementing exercise was also found to be comparable to—if not better than—avoiding coronary artery disease, diabetes, and smoking *combined*.

While there's tremendous value in all the interventions we will discuss, I cannot stress this enough—no other intervention offers this level of protection against premature death and disease. If you were to consider implementing only one intervention from this book, it would be exercise.

HOW EXERCISE TRANSFORMS YOUR BRAIN AND BODY

I'm sure you're aware of how exercise can transform your physical appearance (think bodybuilder versus marathon runner). But the reality is that exercise also transforms the cellular mechanisms inside your body—not just within your muscles, *but in nearly all your organ systems*. I could easily write a book on just this topic alone, because it's that all-encompassing. That said, to give you some perspective, I'd like to highlight a few of the relevant mechanisms as they relate to your health and longevity. This probably comes as no surprise by this point, but many of these processes are highly interrelated.

BRAIN HEALTH AND COGNITIVE FUNCTION

Exercise doesn't just build muscle and strengthen your cardiovascular system. It can quite literally transform your brain at the cellular level, offering benefits that no medication can replicate. All the stuff you've heard about improved mental clarity, mood, focus, and productivity after exercising? There is very real evidence supporting these sentiments, both in the short and long term.

Perhaps the most obvious way that exercise benefits the brain that it directly increases blood flow, immediately delivering more oxygen and nutrients to your neurons. This enhanced blood flow also augments the release of neurotransmitters that improve focus and alertness, which primes your brain for learning in the hours after exercise.

Regular physical activity also stimulates the release of **brain-derived neurotrophic factor (BDNF)**, an incredibly useful protein that acts like fertilizer for your brain cells, promoting neuroplasticity and enhancing your overall cognitive function. BDNF can even increase the volume of key brain regions, particularly your hippocampus—that seahorse-shaped structure crucial for learning and memory formation. Studies have found that consistent physical activity can increase hippocampal volume by approximately 2 percent, *effectively reversing age-related brain tissue loss by one to two years at a time.* That means regular exercise can make a noticeable difference in your memory retention, in addition to improved productivity and focus after a workout.

Exercise also maintains the integrity of your blood-brain barrier, that protective membrane that allows selective passage of certain molecules into your brain while keeping others out. Without exercise, the capillaries that feed the blood-brain barrier can collapse, triggering inflammation and compromising its function. Needless to say, it's best to avoid that.

One last fun fact is the effect of lactate on the brain. You're probably aware of lactate (also less accurately referred to as "lactic acid"), which is commonly associated with the "burn" felt during a hard workout. (Technically, hydrogen ions are responsible for this, not lactate itself, but I'll let it slide.) In medical school, I was taught that this was nothing more than a waste product of anaerobic metabolism, but recently, we've learned that lactate is actually a preferred fuel for your brain, especially during exercise. When you exercise intensely, increased release of lactate into your bloodstream crosses your blood-brain barrier and provides more fuel for your neurons.

By now, we've established that physical health *is* brain health and vice versa. The brain, at the end of the day, is an organ that benefits from exercise just like your heart or muscles—and there is substantial evidence supporting this. Given this clear correlation between exercise, brain health, and mental performance, it should come as no surprise that regular movement can positively impact your mental health, as well.

MENTAL HEALTH AND STRESS REDUCTION

Multiple studies have demonstrated significant improvements in mental health among those who regularly exercise. Physical activity has been shown to reduce symptoms of anxiety and depression at least as effectively as—and in many cases better than—certain medications.

Critically, exercise is also a well-established method for lowering stress by reducing chronically elevated cortisol levels, which ultimately results in lower blood pressure, stabilized blood glucose, and a healthier physiological state. To be clear, cortisol is generally elevated *during* exercise, but avoiding chronic elevations improves overall health—similar to how acute inflammation is largely beneficial while chronic inflammation is not.

Perhaps most valuable for your daily life, exercise promotes better quality deep sleep which enhances your recovery and overall brain function and improves your longevity. We'll cover sleep in depth in Chapter 7, but the main thing to know here is that exercise is a great way to improve the quality of your sleep—particularly morning exercise, if that works for your schedule (and there's even emerging data that intense exercise within four hours of bedtime can actually be harmful to your sleep).

As significant as these benefits for your brain and mental health are, exercise's effects on your body's metabolic systems may be even more critical for extending your lifespan and avoiding the diseases that typically cut lives short, including mood disorders. There is now a field of research and clinical medicine known as metabolic psychiatry, largely pioneered by Harvard psychiatrist Dr. Chris Palmer, which explores the relationship between metabolic and mental health. As strange as this may sound to a conventionally trained provider, it is perhaps of little surprise to you, as we now know how intertwined the mechanisms that underlie disease in your body are and how they relate to your overall physical health.

METABOLIC AND CARDIOVASCULAR HEALTH

At this point, the cardiovascular benefits of exercise are well-documented and largely known. Even still, I think most people aren't *fully* aware of just how dramatic of an impact exercise can have on your metabolic and cardiovascular health.

To briefly touch on some of those benefits, regular physical activity builds stronger heart muscle, maintains blood vessel elasticity, normalizes blood pressure, and decreases resting heart rate. These all independently reduce your risk of heart attack, stroke, and other forms of cardiovascular disease as we discussed in Chapter 2.

Beyond heart health, exercise enhances insulin sensitivity, allowing your cells to extract glucose from your bloodstream more efficiently. This reduces your risk of metabolic syndrome, type 2 diabetes, and the cascade of health problems they trigger. At the cellular level, exercise also significantly reduces inflammation throughout your body, which includes neuroinflammation in the brain. This, as you know, lowers your risk of developing many of the previously mentioned diseases and can slow your rate of cellular aging.

MUSCULOSKELETAL HEALTH AND AGING

As if this all weren't enough, exercise also help maintain your musculoskeletal system, which becomes increasingly important as you age. After age 30, you'll naturally lose about 3–8 percent of your muscle mass per decade, a process that only accelerates after age sixty. This age-related muscle loss, called sarcopenia, can impair your ability to perform even basic tasks like standing, walking, or even carrying groceries, like my friend Jim. Strength training along with adequate protein intake can halt (and in some ways even reverse) this process, maintaining your functional capacity as you age. This is why Jim was able to walk like a thirty-year-old at the age of 88, and he achieved it just by incorporating a few strength-training workouts into his weekly routine!

Similarly, weight-bearing exercise can increase your bone mineral density, thereby reducing your risk of osteoporosis and fractures. Risk of injury from falls can be substantially reduced with stronger bones, muscles, and preserved balance, which can also help you live longer.

If you can believe it, I could have kept going, but I think my editor would have killed me. When you look at all these mechanisms together, there really is no doubt about it—exercise is the closest thing we have to a true anti-aging pill. With that said, I know you're chomping at the bit to get to the "how-to" stuff, so let's get right to it.

Don't feel like you need to write all this down or remember every little detail right now! I've included cheat sheets with all the evidence-based interventions from each intervention chapter at TranscendHealthGroup.com/Resources, where they will also be continually updated as new evidence becomes available.

GETTING STARTED

There are nearly endless approaches to exercise, whether it's hiking along a scenic trail, joining a local pickleball league, taking a dance class, going for a swim, or simply walking your dog around the neighborhood. The simple truth is that *any* level of physical activity, regardless of intensity, is associated with a substantially lower risk of mortality. Rather than overwhelm you with a million options to consider, my approach is to give you a basic framework around how to think about exercise, and most importantly, how to incorporate some form of movement into your daily life.

The best type of exercise is *consistent* exercise that you enjoy and can maintain. Therefore, anything you can do to sustainably build consistent movement into your daily routine will likely be very helpful. This is where your why once again comes into play. With your why in mind, exercise simply becomes another tool at your disposal to help you achieve more of what matters. Instead of feeling like one more thing you "have to do," it becomes an activity that is aligned with who you are and an extension of how you're able to show up best for the world.

That said, maintaining a consistent exercise routine is something that many people struggle with. As we learned in Chapter 1, the cards are stacked against us—our brains have become conditioned to choose the easy way out. But there are a handful of proven techniques that we can use to make this easier. If you've ever struggled to maintain an exercise routine, these are worth knowing about.

MAKE IT EASY

The simplest way to stay consistent with any habit, including exercise, is to make it easy for yourself. In his fantastic book, *Atomic Habits,* James Clear explains how humans gravitate toward the path of least resistance—whether that path produces positive or negative results. For example, if you leave candy out on your counter, you'll naturally eat it because it's within direct eyesight and reach. It's easy. Alternatively, if you keep your treadmill in your basement and every time you use it you have to move a bunch of boxes, wheel it over to the outlet, plug it in, turn it on, and *then* start walking... guess what? You're not going to use it very often. If it's too difficult then there's simply too much resistance around forming that habit, especially when the alternative is something far easier like sitting down on the couch, grabbing the remote, and staying glued to your favorite TV series.

Every step required to get you to the point of exercising is a chance for your brain to resist and take the easy way out. The fewer steps there are, the more likely you are to get to the exercise part and stick with it. Therefore, my advice is to *make it easy for yourself.*

Over the years, I more or less unknowingly created a routine for myself that practically forces me to exercise. I have what is called an early chronotype, which means I tend to wake up early. (About a third of us are wired this way, which we'll cover in Chapter 7.) Between this and the years of conditioning I've undergone through medical training and the military, it is easiest for me to exercise in the morning. But the trick that makes this *really* easy is getting myself ready the night before. This is a routine I initially developed in an effort to not wake my wife—who has more of the "night owl" chronotype—but I quickly realized how much easier it made my life and have stuck with it.

Before I go to bed, I grind my coffee for the next morning (found this one out the hard way) and lay out my supplements, gym clothes, and shoes next to my bed. That way when I wake up, I roll out of bed and literally fall into my routine. It's far easier for me to get ready for the gym than to do anything else. Once I'm dressed, I grab my supplements, coffee, and then just head out—that's it. Not to mention after years of training I know what I have to look forward to, not just while I'm there, but long after. I feel better, stay sharper, and am able to do more of what I love, so I have developed a natural excitement for going, and there's a strong chance you will, too.

It sounds simple and you may have even heard of this trick before, but it really does work. More importantly, it illustrates a crucial point, which is that just a small change to your routine can be profound—we're not talking about heroic effort here. For me, it's as easy as grinding my coffee in advance and having my gym clothes within reach. You may want to think about your routine and identify any areas where you can remove those points of resistance and make it easier for you. The fewer there are, the higher your chances are of consistency and ultimately achieving your goals and your mission.

CREATING A MOVEMENT-CONDUCIVE ENVIRONMENT

One of the best ways to incorporate exercise into your life is to simply set up your environment to be more conducive to regular movement. It has been said that "sitting is the new smoking," and when we look at the data, this statement carries significant weight. Although, to state the obvious, please do not start smoking in favor of sitting....

Your body is designed to move. For tens of thousands of years, your ancestors (here they are again) spent their days walking, running, hunting, gathering food, and building shelters. Like wild animals, there was a time when they were active nearly all day. But in our modern world, many of us spend *eight to ten hours per day* sitting at a desk, in between sitting during our commute, and then even more sitting as we relax in front of the TV at night. This sedentary lifestyle we've unknowingly adopted is a major contributor to many of the health challenges we collectively face.

When you sit for too long, your back muscles and gluteal muscles can lengthen and weaken, your hip flexors can shorten and tighten, your shoulders round forward, and the muscles on the front of your neck shorten and tighten, leading to a condition colloquially known as "tech neck." Over time, prolonged sitting can lead to abnormal spinal anatomy, pinched nerves, decreased flexibility, and poor mobility. It also means you're burning less calories throughout the day, which can lead to weight gain and metabolic syndrome.

If you work from a desk and are able to stand and walk without assistance, I highly recommend considering a standing desk and a walking pad or under-desk treadmill (this is one of the few things in this book I will actually recommend, because there are virtually no downsides). Standing ensures improved spinal posture and activates your antigravity muscles, which are some of the largest muscles in your entire body including your glutes, quads, calves, and paraspinal muscles. Contracting these muscles requires energy, which is why standing burns more calories than sitting—approximately fifty more calories per hour on average, although this varies slightly from person to person.

Under-desk treadmills are another incredible invention that allow you to stay moving while being productive at your desk. You can set a slow pace of just 1–2.5 miles per hour and walk while you work. Before you know it, you'll have accumulated a few miles of walking, and those steps do make a difference. You may have heard of the common goal to achieve 10,000 steps per day for general fitness, and there is plenty of evidence that supports this. According to a large study in the *British Medical Journal* in 2024 that looked at over 72,000 people, walking between 9,000–10,500 steps per day decreased all-cause mortality by 39 percent. That's a substantial risk reduction just from adding more walking to your day—and it can easily be done during your workday with an under-desk treadmill.

Even if you don't work from a desk, there are plenty of other ways to incorporate movement into your daily routine. Maybe you can start riding your bike to work instead of taking the bus. Or when you drive to the grocery store, try parking at the other end of the lot to get a few more steps in both directions. Perhaps try going for a walk next time you need to make a long phone call. Even just setting a timer to remind yourself to get up and move every ninety minutes can be helpful, both for your brain and body. And those breaks are also the perfect time for another one of my favorite activities: exercise snacks!

EXERCISE SNACKS

Another point of resistance that likely affects many people is the belief that if you're not doing a "full" workout you're wasting your time. This couldn't be further from the truth—in fact, even just six minutes of exercise a day could extend your life. Seriously! A 2022 study in the journal *Nature* looked at people who engaged in just two minutes of brief, vigorous activity three times per day and found they had a 38–40 percent reduction in all-cause and cancer mortality, and up to a 49 percent reduction in cardiovascular disease mortality compared to individuals who did not perform the exercises.

If you've ever felt like you're too busy or the idea of an hour-long workout is just too intimidating, exercise snacks are a perfect place to start. All you need are two minutes of high intensity sprint mimickers, such as high-knees-in-place, jumping jacks, air squats, or stair sprints—really, any type of vigorous physical activity will do.

This type of bite-sized exercise is far more impactful than you might think. One way it helps is by releasing **BDNF**, that neurotransmitter we discussed earlier which improves blood glucose regulation, impacting your metabolic health (among other things). Low levels of BDNF are also associated with an array of neurodegenerative and neuroinflammatory disorders, whereas higher levels are associated with improved memory and cognitive function.

If you work at home or in an office, these exercise snacks can also help you feel more alert and focused during the day due to increased blood flow to your brain and an increase in neurotransmitters such as epinephrine, norepinephrine, and dopamine. If you ever feel sluggish midday, especially after a big meal, this is a great strategy to consider.

If this is of interest, performing them throughout your workday, ideally just before or after meals, can have the greatest impact.

To make it easy and sustainable, start with one around lunch time. Once that habit sticks, you can then add more into your routine. As a bonus, when you begin to notice the performance benefits, the reward circuits in your brain will help you crave them more, thereby increasing the chance that you'll keep at it. Is your why worth six minutes? I'd bet I can guess your answer.

NO GYM? NO PROBLEM

One further point of resistance for many people is the idea that they have to go to a gym or spend thousands of dollars on fancy equipment to build out a home gym. There are *plenty* of other ways to exercise that don't involve any equipment whatsoever. Most importantly, if you don't like the idea of going to a gym or it's not convenient for you, you don't have to! Remember our first rule: make it easy! Exercising should be fun, and if lifting weights or going to a gym sounds like torture to you, that's a sign of major resistance and you might want to look for a different activity. Body weight exercises like push-ups, pull-ups, planks, wall-sits, lunges, air-squats, sit-ups, and yoga are all viable solutions that can get you into incredible shape.

Most forms of cardiovascular exercise also don't require any (or at least very minimal) equipment. Things like running, hiking, walking, jogging, jumping jacks, jump rope, high-knees, and burpees can provide ample cardiorespiratory fitness. If you happen to have access to a bicycle, elliptical, or rower, these can also be great low-impact methods too.

Outside of the aforementioned, anything that gets you moving is great. If you enjoy playing a certain sport, maybe this is a sign to look for a rec league. If you dread exercise, that just means you need to find a different form that works for you.

THE THREE EXERCISE PILLARS

While simply focusing on consistent physical movement is an effective strategy to incorporate exercise into your life, for those looking to go a bit deeper, there are ultimately three dedicated types of exercise that have been shown to improve your health and longevity: cardiovascular training, strength training, and high intensity interval training (HIIT).

The evidence indicates that a proper exercise routine should probably include these three pillars.

EXERCISE PILLAR #1: CARDIOVASCULAR TRAINING

If you want to live a long, healthy life, cardiovascular training really can't be overlooked. Given our basic understanding of the cardiovascular system and cardiovascular disease, by now I hope it's easy to see why this might be the case. A stronger cardiovascular system means more blood is able to flow freely and deliver key nutrients to all corners of your body, keeping your various organ systems operating well and slowing your rate of cellular aging in the process.

You can easily make exercise productive by listening to a podcast, having a walking meeting, or reading a book. I regularly pre-select podcasts before I leave for the gym and sometimes read medical journals or research topics that interest me in between sets. (I'm a nerd, I know.)

Cardiovascular training conditions your aerobic Type 1 muscle fibers, which are heavily dependent on oxygen for their metabolism. In doing so, this raises the population of mitochondria within your cells, which help to maintain your energy balance and improve your blood glucose regulation and metabolic efficiency (among many other things). All of this ultimately translates to a lowered risk of developing cardiovascular disease, cancer, infection, and ultimately lowering all-cause mortality, to name a few.

According to the evidence, if you want to optimize your brain health and longevity, you should aim for a total of about 200 minutes of cardiovascular activity per week. This should ideally take place in sessions of 60–75 minutes, three to four times per week (or more if you are more conditioned).

There are five heart rate "zones" within cardiovascular training, with Zone 2 training being particularly important given its activation of these benefits, although there is data that supports spending some time in each zone depending on your personal goals. Zone 2 is defined as the point at which maximum fat burning in your body occurs and is considered relatively low-intensity work.

One way to think about this would be training at approximately 60–70 percent of your maximum heart rate, which you can measure on many cardiovascular machines or with a wearable device. If you don't have access to equipment that can measure your heart rate, here's a quick guide to the five zones based on another metric called your RPE or "rate of perceived exertion," which exists on a scale from 1–10 with 1 representing the least amount of effort and 10 being all-out maximum effort:

- **In Zone 1**, you're recovering, more or less breathing normally, and still able to hold a conversation with ease. RPE: 1–2
- **In Zone 2**, you're breathing heavily but still be able to hold a conversation—albeit, not as easily. RPE: 3–4

- **In Zone 3**, you're breathing moderately hard. Conversation is possible, but requires much more effort. RPE: 5–6
- **In Zone 4**, you're breathing very hard, and it is extremely difficult to hold a conversation. RPE: 7–8
- **In Zone 5**, you're giving maximum effort and conversation is not possible. RPE: 9–10

Whatever method you prefer, as the timeless Nike slogan encourages us, just do it: running, jogging, cycling, elliptical, rowing, swimming. Keep in mind that cross-training, or mixing up the type of exercise you are doing, can also reduce the risk of injury from overtraining.

EXERCISE PILLAR #2: STRENGTH TRAINING

Occasionally when I'm explaining the value of exercise to a patient, they'll tell me they don't like lifting weights. My half-joking response is, "Would you like to die sooner?"

While most people are aware of the health benefits of cardiovascular exercise, I find the general public is often misinformed on the benefits of strength training. Lifting weights or any type of general resistance training is not just for men who want to show off their muscles or athletes looking to push themselves to the next level, and it's certainly not solely for superficial gain. The benefits of strength training are considerable, and they become *even more invaluable* as we age.

Once my older patients recover from the shock of my terrible jokes, I'll often share a crucial statistic: in patients over sixty, the one-year mortality rate after a hip fracture is 14–58 percent. And critically, the people at highest risk for hip fracture are those who have low musculoskeletal strength, impaired balance, and low bone mineral density. Dedicated strength training helps improve all those metrics, making it particularly important for elderly people.

Strength training focuses on the activation of anaerobic or glycolytic Type 2 muscle fibers, which primarily use glucose for fuel. When these fibers atrophy and eventually die, they cannot regenerate, potentially leading to the previously mentioned condition sarcopenia—the age-related muscle loss that significantly impairs basic functions like standing, walking, and carrying groceries. Fortunately, these fibers can be maintained through strength training. As you age, maintaining muscle is incredibly important to not only prevent sarcopenia and minimize your risk of injury from falls, but also to maintain your metabolism.

Strength training increases your lean mass, or the percentage of your body that is made up of muscle. Muscle is very metabolically active, so the more muscle you have, the more calories you burn at rest—another 6–10 calories per day per pound of muscle in fact, which helps you maintain a healthy lean-to-fat mass ratio.

To break this down, let's say you gained just five pounds of muscle after starting regular strength training (not a heroic feat or at all uncommon). Using just 6 calories per day, that would equate to burning an additional 900 calories per month or 10,800 calories per year *at rest*, which equates to over 3 pounds of fat loss without you doing anything! (For context, it takes about 3,500 calories of energy burned to lose one pound of fat.) Of course, doing the work to gain and maintain that muscle in the first place also burns calories, but the point is this quickly becomes a positive feedback loop in terms of you gaining strength, which decreases your risk of injury, which adds muscle, which burns more energy, which decreases your storage of additional fat, which decreases your risk of disease, which helps you live longer, and so on.

When it comes to your brain health, strength training also provides similar benefits to cardiovascular training. It can also provide a substantial increase in the delivery of lactate to your brain along with increased blood flow and all the benefits that we covered above. But critically, strength training also releases signaling molecules from your muscles and your bones. Myokines (a class of cytokine) like cathepsin B can cross the blood-brain barrier, further increasing BDNF and activating another protein called PGC-1α, which increases mitochondrial production, further improving your energy metabolism and enhancing critical cellular processes like autophagy.

During strength training, your bones release a hormone called osteocalcin, which can also cross the blood-brain barrier and act on your hippocampus to improve memory and learning, reduce symptoms of anxiety and depression, and even protect against age-related cognitive decline. Preliminary data even suggests increased osteocalcin levels might improve outcomes after stroke by promoting neuronal survival. And finally, strength training has also been demonstrated to substantially improve mood with multiple studies showing a consistent reduction in depressive symptoms, anxiety, and overall cognitive stress.

There are *many* ways to achieve an effective strength training program, including bodyweight exercises, machines, free weights, resistance bands, kettlebells, and TRX bands. Whatever methods you choose, you'll ideally want to aim for two to four training sessions per week focused on compound movements. You should also be sure to incorporate all major muscle groups to avoid imbalance, which can predispose you to injury.

If you are new to strength training, working with a professional such as a personal trainer is a highly effective way to start, although it can be costly. There are also endless free resources on YouTube and online. Nowadays, there are tons of exercise apps that practically mimic a personal trainer, providing customized workouts based on your goals.

EXERCISE PILLAR #3: HIGH INTENSITY INTERVAL TRAINING

The last pillar of exercise is most commonly known as high intensity interval training, or "HIIT" for short. This type of training involves short bursts of intense effort followed by periods of rest. HIIT workouts confer multiple benefits and should likely be part of any standard exercise program due to their unique impact on brain health and a measurable parameter known as your **VO_2 max**. For the uninitiated, VO_2 max is defined as the maximal oxygen consumption that your body can utilize during exercise and it is a key longevity metric. It's essentially an indirect measurement of your mitochondrial function, which is where your aerobic metabolism takes place. And as you know, healthy mitochondria help you live longer.

The actual measurement signifies the maximum amount of oxygen that your body can consume per kilogram of body weight per minute of intense physical activity. The ranges are rather broad and decline with age, but a thirty-five-year-old in "fair" shape may have a VO_2 max of 30 mL/kg/min, whereas it may be closer to 45 mL/kg/min in someone the same age in "excellent" shape. Similarly, "fair" for a sixty-five-year-old may be closer to 23 mL/kg/min and "excellent" in the 35 mL/kg/min range, just to give you an idea.

The point is, the higher your VO_2 max, the more effective your body is at supplying blood to your muscles and the more efficient your muscles are at extracting that oxygen from your blood. It is a great indicator of overall fitness, and a high VO_2 max has been strongly correlated with a longer lifespan and improved brain health. While your VO_2 max does typically decrease with age, as noted above, staying in the upper range for your age bracket is largely within your control, and just one to two HIIT workouts per week are typically enough to do that.

You can generate precise measurements of your VO_2 max in an exercise physiology lab, although this may not be entirely necessary depending on your specific health goals. This typically involves wearing a heart rate monitor and a sealed mask to record how much oxygen you absorb and how much carbon dioxide you're exhaling while running on a treadmill or doing some type of intense aerobic activity. You can also conduct a rudimentary version of this test with apps and wearables like the Oura Ring or a six-minute walking test, where you walk as far as you can as quickly as you can without jogging or running and the app provides a rough estimate based upon the distance you were able to cover within that time frame.

Achieving a higher VO_2 max helps with just about everything in your body, but it's particularly relevant to your brain—which should come as no surprise given the fact that your brain receives 20 percent of your blood supply, as we've covered. A higher VO_2 max has been shown to increase the thickness of your cerebral cortex, which, as you may recall, is the gray matter on the outer portion of your brain where the majority of your neurons live.

In particular, your frontal and temporal lobes appear to receive a substantial boost, as well as your cingulate cortex and hippocampus. Elevated VO_2 max measurements have also been associated with improved white matter integrity, which can improve the efficiency of communication between your brain networks that otherwise slow with aging. All this translates to improved cognitive function, executive function, memory, processing speed, cognitive reserve, and mental resilience.

According to a 2022 *JAMA* study looking at over 122,000 people, "elite" level performance—defined as those in the top 2.5 percent of VO_2 max measurements compared with the lowest performers—was associated with an *80 percent reduction in all-cause mortality risk*. To put that into perspective, that risk reduction was comparable to if not better than avoiding coronary artery disease, diabetes, and smoking *combined*. Similarly, a 2018 *AHA* study looking at sixty-one participants in their late forties to early fifties, found their apparent heart age decreased by an average of *twenty years* after undergoing a vigorous VO_2 max-enhancing exercise protocol for two years!

As mentioned previously, increasing your VO_2 max can be achieved with just one to two HIIT workouts per week. It should be noted that this type of training is on the more advanced end of the exercise spectrum—in other words, if you're starting to train for the first time, this is very likely something you'll need to work up to. However, once you establish a baseline level of conditioning, they will by definition remain challenging but doable.

The most common HIIT-type sessions tend to be done in a class setting. Most gyms will offer some options for this and there are nearly endless apps, YouTube videos, and online programs that you can follow along with from the comfort of your own home. For the most part, all you need for these workouts is an exercise mat and some room to move around. HIIT exercises can include things like sprints, burpees, mountain climbers, squat jumps, jumping jacks, high knees, lunge jumps, pushups, and more.

For those who would rather create their own program than attend a class, there are many options. If you're looking for more information on these, I've included a PDF with some examples on the resource page, at TranscendHealthGroup.com/Resources. The specific type of HIIT exercises you choose to do aren't particularly important; the key is to work them into your training program and stick with them. If nothing else, it will at least make all other forms of exercise feel substantially easier.

By the way, remember that magic longevity pill? If you create a training program that includes each of these three pillars and stick with it consistently, then congratulations! You've just found the magic pill that will not only increase your lifespan and your healthspan but makes everything easier along the way. Plus, you'll very likely look and feel great in the process!

ADHERENCE

I was never the biggest or most athletic kid growing up, but I was always active. I played everything from football to soccer to tennis and track. (I even tried basketball at one point, but that ended quickly.) In high school, I was a competitive rower, and in college I played rugby for a few semesters—about which my doctor once rightly asked me, "What is wrong with you?" While those activities kept me in relatively good shape, they don't come close to the level of consistency and intensity of exercise I experienced during my time in the Navy.

One of my most cherished memories is of a dark morning in Newport, Rhode Island...

When I close my eyes, I am instantly transported back. The air is cool, the faint Newport fog hovers above the ground, and all I can hear is the rhythmic cadence of 150 feet striking the pavement in unison. Then, the distinct, melodic call from Chief Petty Officer Ruiz.

"C-130 ROLLIN' DOWN THE STRIP!"

Our entire company echoes him in perfect unison.

"O-D-S GONNA TAKE A LITTLE TRIP!"

Our words reverberate off the barracks and fade into the distance as we jog, the sun faintly cresting above the horizon. I literally get goosebumps every time I think about it.

In the summer of 2013, this was my daily routine during my time at the United States Navy's Officer Training Command. Wake up, make bed, dress for PT, and be outside in formation in no time, ready for our daily morning session. Some days it was a 5K group run, others it was pushups, sit-ups, sprints, and plyometrics. Since we would be done before most people had even woken up, after chow and a full day of classroom lectures, I would go lift weights in the afternoons with a few of my other "gym bros." To be twenty-five again...

Regular exercise is mandatory for any active duty soldier in the US military, not only because we need fit people to defend our country, but because the government understands the positive health implications. Whether you like it or not, when you join the US military you become government property—and the government wants to keep their property in good working order. That's why I, as a neurologist, was still required to exercise, not to mention learn how to patch leaks on a sinking ship and put out fires in a full SCBA and flameproof gear as if I were on the front lines. In the eyes of the US government, Chief Ruiz waking me up every morning to run three miles at 4:00 a.m. was akin to an aircraft mechanic doing routine maintenance on a fighter plane (which, ironically, is where Chief spent his career before training us). It was just something that needed to happen to keep things working properly.

In your life, you don't need to have a Chief Ruiz, which you should be thankful for (our parting encounter was him making me roll in a sand pit just hours before my graduation). But you do need to adhere to a consistent exercise program. Given our focus on evidence-based interventions, it would only make sense to look at what the evidence says, and the research demonstrates several key factors that improve your adherence to any fitness program.

The first is belief in yourself. It turns out that self-belief in your ability to succeed in a specific activity substantially improves the likelihood that you stick with your training program and achieve your desired outcome. Becoming aware of your own capabilities has also been shown to improve adherence to a given exercise program.

So, before you embark upon your exercise journey, think back to your why and visualize the outcome you want to achieve. The more specific the better.

How do you look in the future? How is your body different than it is now? What are you able to do? How much weight are you able to lift? How far can you run? For how long? How much mentally sharper do you feel? How is your energy? How do you feel? Now that you have that in focus, you just need to *believe* that it is going to happen—which it will, if you stick with it.

If you're feeling skeptical, there's plenty of neuroscience behind why this works. Visualization activates the same neural pathways as actually performing the activity itself, essentially priming your brain and body for success. This is a technique that elite athletes, pilots, and Formula 1 drivers use regularly to improve their performance. If you're curious, go look up a video of Sergio Perez driving the Mexican Grand Prix blind. He isn't actually driving blind, but moving a steering wheel with his eyes closed while a video of him driving plays in the background. He can visualize the track so well that his movements sync up perfectly with the video, as he completes every turn and gear change with precision. This mental practice helps create the motor programs and muscle memory that allow these elite athletes to perform at such high levels, but it can also be used in everyday situations.

The second factor is technology. In a meta-analysis of older adults who underwent an exercise program, the group exposed to technology as a way to enhance or assist their workouts had over a 91 percent adherence to the program. One way technology can help is by "gamifying" exercise, making it less of a chore and more of a fun activity. Many of the at-home exercise systems like Peloton and Tonal provide scoreboards and achievements, while wearable devices can track your progress and even let you compete against friends in fitness competitions. While technology won't solve all your problems, there is certainly evidence showing it can be an effective tool in adhering to your exercise program. We'll talk more about this in Chapter 10.

The last factor is to get in a group setting. Supervised group-based exercise has been demonstrated as an effective way to increase adherence to an exercise program. For centuries, athletes around the world have utilized this concept from training for the Olympic games in ancient Greece to present day little league. The camaraderie of a team, reliance on one another, desire to not let one another down, and sacrificing your personal comfort for the benefit of the group all have ancient human roots in our social development. If you are currently or have ever been on any sort of team, you'll know exactly what I'm talking about. Physical activity is far more fun and certainly more motivating this way, and a large part of why I still get chills thinking about morning group PT in Rhode Island.

To be clear, this doesn't need to involve joining a sports team or putting yourself in some hyper-competitive environment, either. Many people find motivation in simply exercising with a group of like-minded people who share similar goals. Whether it's a walking group, yoga, or even an online fitness community—being surrounded by others who are also trying to improve their health has been shown to make a significant difference in consistency.

If you're having trouble sticking to a training program, you may want to look at how you can shake things up to incorporate one or even all three of these elements. The first step should always be to get back to your why and visualize the desired outcome you want to achieve—and I don't just mean your physical results, but who or what you're doing all of this for. Your why isn't just something to be written down and forgotten about, it should be your daily motivator. That, plus the scope of knowledge you now have around why exercise is valuable should make your adherence much easier.

And remember: whatever you do, *make it fun!* You should enjoy your time being active. Life's too short to spend thirty minutes or an hour every day doing something you hate, and that's certainly a recipe for failure anyway. If you don't currently enjoy your exercise routine, I'd urge you to experiment until you find something you love. Maybe that means exercising with a training partner, joining a class, finding a recreational sports team, or "gamifying" your exercise with a wearable device.

Keep in mind that, above all else, what's most important is simply incorporating movement into your life. You don't need to have a strict, regimented routine if it doesn't align with your goals. Movement can be spontaneous and joyful—as simple as dancing with your kids, gardening, taking calls while walking, playing tag in the backyard, or even doing squats while brushing your teeth. It all counts, and your body doesn't care whether you're doing pull-ups or chasing your friends around the yard—it just wants to move.

KEY TAKEAWAYS

1. **Exercise is the single most powerful longevity intervention available to you.** Regular physical activity can reduce your risk of dying from any cause by up to 40 percent, decrease your chances of developing dementia by 40 percent, and cut your risk of heart attack and stroke by 38 percent. No other intervention offers this level of protection against premature death and disease.

2. **A complete exercise program includes three essential pillars:** Cardiovascular training, strength training, and high-intensity interval training (HIIT). Each type of exercise activates different beneficial pathways in your body.

3. **Consistency trumps intensity.** The best exercise program is one you can stick with long-term. Make exercise easy by removing points of resistance, creating a movement-conducive environment, and connecting your workouts to your why. Even small amounts of movement, like two-minute "exercise snacks," provide significant benefits if done consistently over time.

You can find a list of all the specific interventions from this chapter in the Exercise Cheat Sheet at TranscendHealthGroup.com/Resources.

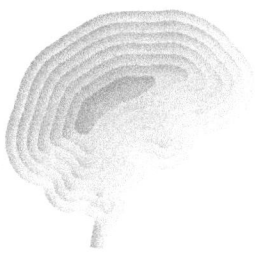

CHAPTER 6
NUTRITION

A LOT OF PEOPLE think nutrition is the easy part. Just eat "clean," right? But what I've seen again and again, both in the Navy and in my civilian medical practice, is that even the most disciplined people often struggle here. Not because they lack willpower or motivation, but because nutrition is more emotionally and environmentally complex than we give it credit for.

In a technical sense, food is fuel for your body. But in reality, food is much more than that—it's emotional, social, and habitual. It's tied to our sense of safety, the reward system in our brains, and the cultures we live in. It's connected to childhood memories and family traditions. For many, it's how we cope with stress. And unlike exercise, where the effort is concentrated and visible, nutritional choices happen dozens of times throughout the day, often unconsciously.

Snacks, takeout, a night out to dinner, treating yourself after a stressful day at work—it's often seemingly invisible moments like these that add up to throw off even the most well-intentioned nutrition plans. This is not to say that everyone must follow an extremely strict nutrition plan, but that the cards are once again stacked against us. Between our busy lives, an overabundance of processed foods, and a seemingly endless flow of misinformation, it is only natural to fall into this trap.

When I was an active duty Navy physician stationed at Camp Lejeune Naval Medical Center, I would regularly have conversations with sailors who were seemingly doing everything "right" but still struggling to get control of their weight.

"Doc, I just don't know what to do. I'm eating super clean, I run four miles a day, and I go to group PT after that. They put me on FEP and I'm going to get passed over for a promotion again."

FEP, which is the Navy's Fitness Enhancement Program, is a rigorous exercise and nutrition plan designed to help out-of-shape sailors return to Navy fitness regulations. While data on the program is not readily available to the public, several articles boast a success rate of over 90 percent. Given what I've seen of the program, I would believe that; however, I still frequently worked alongside sailors that were struggling to regain control of their health while on this program.

According to a public report given by Navy Admiral and former Chief of Naval Operations, Lisa Franchetti, to the Senate in 2023, 68 percent of active duty service members are overweight or obese. This isn't terribly different from the 74 percent of the general American population that meets the same criteria, although it is surprising given the relatively young age of most active duty service members and the rigorous training they're forced to endure.

So, what is really holding back these sailors, even when they are placed on a strict nutrition plan? The reality is that the military can't control every single calorie they consume, and they were likely snacking or going off their nutrition plan in ways that were seemingly insignificant but collectively hindered their progress.

There are many reasons why people struggle to control their weight, but a central component is *proper* adherence to a *proper* nutrition plan. It's easy to feel like you're eating the right things, but without a basic knowledge of what—and critically, how much—to put into your body, it's very easy to overconsume by snacking or consuming energy-dense but nutrient-poor calories. Like exercise, adhering to a nutrition plan can be challenging—but it can be made easy with the right motivation (your why) and a basic understanding of how the food you're eating impacts your body and your health.

In this chapter, we'll explore how nutrition affects your body, how it relates to aging, and what you need to know to create a nutrition plan that works for you. The goal, as always, is to develop a plan that is sustainable long-term. Small changes here can make a big difference over time, and one simple change to shift your mindset around food is to embrace the simple idea that *you are what you eat*.

YOU ARE WHAT YOU EAT

The phrase "you are what you eat" is a very accurate way to sum up the importance of your nutrition. Quite literally, you are composed of the very molecules you have once eaten. On average, you are an entirely new "person" every seven years, meaning you have replaced your old building blocks with new ones—and those new ones come from the foods you consume.

The rate of replacement varies depending on the type of tissue in question, but just as an example, your muscle turns over at a rate of about 1–2 percent per day. This means that every 50–100 days, you have completely broken down and rebuilt all of the muscle in your entire body. The lining of your intestines, on the other hand, completely replaces itself every three to five days. And, most impressive to me, your brain recycles all of its protein every nine days! That blows my mind, no pun intended.

The food you consume is where you obtain all of your key building blocks: the proteins and amino acids that make up your muscles and bones, the healthy fats that make up various parts of your brain and nervous system, the micronutrients that serve as cofactors for the millions of reactions happening in your cells every second, and the glucose that can generate ATP, the energy currency in your body. Many have said this in one way or another, but I love Dr. Mark Hyman's mantra that "food is medicine." It's true, and what you eat matters.

I often tell my patients, "You wouldn't put diesel in a gasoline engine." The same principle applies to your body. You're designed to operate well on certain fuels and not others.

With that in mind, the key to improving your nutrition is to create a plan that provides your body with the correct fuels in the correct amounts, but one that also integrates well into your lifestyle. A nutrition plan is not a "one size fits all" prescription. We all have unique genetic differences, allergies, caloric needs, personal goals, health conditions, preferences, and beliefs—all of which should be taken into consideration before creating a personalized nutrition plan.

This is one reason why I don't love the term *diet*. To me, it confers the idea of limiting oneself or generally doing something unpleasant. It also implies a limited timeframe, suggesting that it is a means to an end in order to achieve a specific outcome such as losing 15 pounds or getting in shape for beach season. This indirectly implies that once it's over, you can go right back to what you were doing before—which is obviously what got you to where you don't want to be in the first place.

Instead, I would look at food for what it is: an investment in your future self and a lever that will move you closer to achieving your why. I eat healthy foods because they are aligned with my purpose and my overall goals in life, not because someone told me to. It does not feel like a chore for me to eat a salad over French fries; it feels natural. It's motivating because I know that each bite is helping me make progress toward what I want to achieve in life.

That underlying motivation combined with a general knowledge of what to eat and in what quantities will serve you far better than any diet ever could. So, that will be our focus.

ADHERENCE TO NUTRITION

Nutrition is very similar to exercise in that small, incremental changes you make now can pay dividends in the future while also improving your daily life in the meantime. The key here is consistency, which brings us back to that word from the last chapter—*adherence*.

Just like crafting an exercise plan that you love will be far more fruitful than forcing yourself to do something you hate, the goal should be to craft a nutrition plan that suits you. Adherence to a proper nutrition plan has been shown to be a valuable long-term predictor of successful weight loss in various studies where people were even prescribed exactly the same food. This might sound intuitive, but it highlights the importance of finding a healthy nutrition plan that you can actually stick with.

So, how can you stick to your nutrition plan once it's created? For starters, having a clear why will provide a significant advantage. But given the current evidence available, there are a few things we know can also make it easier:

1. **Tailor your nutrition plan to your personal preferences.** While you still should focus on meeting specific nutritional goals, your plan should be suited to your preferences so you're able to maintain it long-term.

2. **Control the drive to eat via hunger suppression.** Strategies like intermittent fasting, exercise, ketosis, moderate use of caffeine, adequate sleep, and stress management all play important roles here. There's plenty of evidence that these strategies work, which we'll discuss later on.
3. **Make it fun.** Rather than feeling like a chore, healthy cooking and eating can be fun. Use it as a chance to get creative and enjoy good food with friends or loved ones.
4. **Make it social.** The familial bonding you can achieve from eating in groups you regularly socialize with has also been demonstrated to lower stress, which we know is valuable for your longevity.
5. **View nutrition as medicine and fuel for your body.** You can literally heal yourself with food. If you want your body to perform optimally for the long haul, you want to be made of the best parts—that mental shift alone can be incredibly motivating.
6. **Learn about nutrition.** Educating yourself on the basics of healthy eating is essential, as this will help you craft a nutrition plan customized to your needs. Learn how to read food labels, especially the ingredients, and understand exactly what you are putting in your body.

As an example of how some of these can be worked into a nutrition plan, I'll give you some insight into how I eat. To be clear, this does not mean you should follow the same pattern; I just want you to observe the principles and intentionality behind what I choose and why.

I am an omnivore, meaning I eat both plant and animal-based foods because I have found this to be the most sustainable long-term plan for me. I practice intermittent fasting and drink black coffee in the morning because it helps suppress my appetite and, along with exercise, controls my hunger until it's time for my first meal of the day around 11:00 AM. Most of what I consume are plant-based whole foods with a heavy focus on a variety of fresh vegetables, greens, salads, fiber, muesli, nuts, berries, and olive oil. However, I also regularly consume fish and Greek yogurt to ensure adequate protein intake, with the occasional steak maybe once or twice a month or a burger if I really want to treat myself.

I fortunately married an amazing cook, so she does most of the preparation of our food, but I often get asked to play sous chef, which makes the experience more enjoyable and memorable for both of us. We also regularly dine out, either together for a personal date night or with friends and family, which creates a warm experience around food. I do my best to make informed decisions about what I order, where we shop, and what I choose to put in my body, because I know doing so either enhances my health and performance or hinders it, which positively or negatively impacts my mission to help more people live longer, healthier, and more impactful lives.

I do not follow a rigorous nutrition plan down to the calorie or macronutrient, but I'm able to use my knowledge of nutrition to make informed decisions about what I eat on a daily basis to maintain a healthy lean mass and ensure I am receiving adequate amounts of macro and micronutrients. What I can't achieve through food, I supplement, which we'll cover in Chapter 8.

That, combined with some of the adherence techniques above and the knowledge that each meal I eat supports my why makes eating healthy nearly effortless and seamlessly integrated into my life. Once this clicks into place, you'll likely experience a similar ease as your own habits begin to align more with what matters most to you. Over time, making the "right" choices only feels more natural and easier.

WHAT HAPPENS WHEN YOU EAT?

You know that food is essential fuel for your body, but what's really happening when you eat? To create a useful framework for thinking about your nutrition, it's helpful to broadly understand what's happening biologically when you consume a given type of food and how it might impact your longevity.

At a very high level, there are two critical biochemical pathways in your body that are directly affected by your food intake. The first is called **AMPK (Adenosine Monophosphate-Activated Protein Kinase)** and the second is known as **mTOR (Mechanistic or Mammalian Target of Rapamycin).**

I have to say that the upcoming descriptions are grossly oversimplified. These pathways are incredibly nuanced, interconnected, and the full scope of their effects are still not fully understood. I will include some of the finer details later, but for now, it's just important that you understand the big picture.

Remember earlier when I said that your DNA is constantly being damaged and repaired? Well, that same concept essentially applies to your entire body. Imagine your body as a city that's constantly under construction. New buildings are constantly being put up while old ones are torn down, and their materials recycled. This never truly "ends."

Of course, this is a metaphor and there are no buildings in your body—really, we're talking about the constant creation of new building blocks and the recycling of old ones. We've already discussed some of these mechanisms, like autophagy, but there are many more that aren't worth specifying for our purposes here—just know they do exist.

Think of the AMPK pathway like your body's maintenance and recycling department, which is constantly tearing down old buildings and recycling their parts. mTOR, on the other hand, is the construction and storage department—it is responsible for the construction of new buildings, as well as organizing and storing all the extra materials for future projects.

These two pathways go hand in hand. For your body to continue to function optimally and age well, they need to be in balance, and that balance is achieved largely through your nutrition plan. AMPK and mTOR are turned on or off based on a number of conditions, but chief among them is the food that enters your body—what you eat, how much, and when. Much like how those construction and waste removal departments might be called in more or less frequently depending on the amount of building materials and money that flow into the city.

While this construction and waste removal analogy is a conceptually useful way to think of this, it is worth going a bit deeper into the biochemistry of how these two pathways function and how your nutrition affects them. I promise I'll keep the jargon to a minimum.

AMPK (ADENOSINE MONOPHOSPHATE-ACTIVATED PROTEIN KINASE)

AMPK is essentially a survival mechanism that becomes activated when your body undergoes any sort of external pressure like physical stress (exercise) or going without food for a period of time. Your body doesn't know what's coming next—it doesn't know if you'll be exercising for hours on end or fasting for days—so it tells the rest of your cells to brace for impact and start cleaning house, become more energy-conscious, and release your "back-up" stores of energy.

In simple terms, AMPK:

- Helps clean up old cellular junk through autophagy
- Improves energy efficiency by improving your mitochondrial function
- Signals your body to burn fat rather than store it
- Helps maintain healthy blood sugar levels by helping your tissues better utilize it
- Enhances your cells' resistance to stress and oxidative damage
- Overall is associated with longer lifespan and healthy aging

For the scientifically inclined, AMPK increases **catabolism**, which is the breakdown of components like muscle and protein, and decreases **anabolism**, which is the building of these same components. It downregulates the mTOR pathway—meaning it gets turned on less frequently—and decreases protein synthesis and fat storage. It also decreases cholesterol and fatty acid synthesis, lowers blood glucose levels, and increases glucose utilization within your body.

Perhaps what's most relevant is that upregulation of AMPK—turning it on more frequently—has been linked with a longer lifespan in model organisms, and therefore, with increased longevity. To be clear, there are not an abundance of robust human studies that support this *yet*; however, there appears to be a fair amount of information supporting increased longevity in the setting of mTOR inhibition (covered below), which by definition also upregulates AMPK. In practical terms, however, this is all naturally achieved through proper nutrition and exercise.

mTOR (MECHANISTIC OR MAMMALIAN TARGET OF RAPAMYCIN)

mTOR is the major building and storage pathway in your body, which becomes activated when resources are plentiful—particularly after eating protein-rich foods, in particular animal-based protein, and with insulin secretion after ingesting carbohydrates. A variety of other hormone signaling pathways, including testosterone, IGF-1 (insulin-like growth factor 1), and others also turn on mTOR, but are outside the scope of this discussion.

In simple terms, mTOR:

- Instructs your body to build new proteins and muscle
- Promotes storage of energy as adipose tissue, or fat
- Becomes activated after meals rich in animal protein and carbohydrates
- Is necessary for recovery and repair
- Helps build strength and muscle

To go a bit deeper on how this all works, mTOR increases protein synthesis in your body, which makes up most of your visible structure. It is activated by the BCAAs (branched-chain amino acids), which come largely from animal-based protein. It is also activated by insulin, the fat storage hormone, and arginine, another amino acid.

Basically, mTOR activation inhibits autophagy and the breakdown of protein, essentially turning off the recycling mechanisms in favor of building new parts of your body and storing energy.

THE BALANCING ACT

At the risk of angering my scientific colleagues, I'd say it's fair to think about mTOR and AMPK as sort of opposites—mTOR builds while AMPK conserves. Both of them are necessary for your survival, but they need to be kept in balance. When one becomes more active than the other for long periods of time, problems can occur.

In today's world, overactivation of mTOR is a primary concern. When mTOR is perpetually turned on, it leads to an excess energy imbalance, resulting in increased storage, inflammation, obesity, and nearly all of the metabolic issues and chronic diseases we previously covered, which ultimately translates to increased morbidity and a shortened lifespan.

Much of this is due to overeating. When you consume more calories than your body needs, mTOR gets turned on and your body stores all that additional energy, largely in the form of fat, for a rainy day. That would be of minimal concern if you were to subsequently engage in an extended bout of physical activity or go for a long time without eating, which is what that mechanism is designed for. However, because most people today lead largely sedentary lifestyles and have food readily available at all times, that "rainy day" never comes—which leads to the subsequent predictable weight gain, obesity, and disease patterns.

Overactivation of AMPK can be problematic as well, as it can lead to accelerated loss of lean mass, notably muscle, loss of strength, increased susceptibility to disease, immune system dysfunction, and premature death. That said, this is probably not a major concern for *most* people.

The point is the type and quantity of food coming into your body can largely dictate when these pathways get turned on, which means this is—ready for it?—*largely within your control*. Here is a general list of strategies that activate each.

Foods and practices that activate AMPK (the recycling department):
- Fasting or time-restricted eating (going 12–16 or more hours without food)
- Exercise, particularly high-intensity or endurance training
- Foods rich in polyphenols, like berries, dark chocolate, green tea, and olive oil
- Foods containing resveratrol, like grapes (not wine), blueberries, and pistachios
- Staying in a slight caloric deficit (consuming fewer calories than you burn)
- Consuming fermented foods like yogurt, kimchi, or sauerkraut

Foods and practices that activate mTOR (the building and storage department):
- Protein-rich meals, especially those high in animal proteins and dairy
- Foods rich in branched-chain amino acids (BCAAs), like beef, chicken, fish, eggs, and whey protein
- Consuming excess calories beyond what your body needs
- Eating frequently throughout the day (constant grazing or snacking)
- High insulin levels from consuming refined carbohydrates and sugar (not recommended)

Given this basic knowledge, you can see how relatively simple changes around your nutritional habits can manipulate the activation of either pathway. If your goal were to lower mTOR and activate AMPK (like most people), then you might want to avoid snacking and focus on consuming fewer (but high-quality) calories overall. You may also want to experiment with intermittent fasting, if that works for you. Swapping out animal-based proteins for plant-based options might also be a good idea. Reducing your overall calorie count and working in some fermented foods could be helpful. These are merely examples to get you thinking about what might work for you and could serve as a sustainable regimen.

If you do want to lower AMPK and activate mTOR—maybe you're a bodybuilder looking to pack on muscle—then you might want to focus on more animal-based, protein rich meals and consider consuming excess calories. That said, if you're a bodybuilder you probably don't need me to tell you this and have a far more in-depth understanding of your training and nutritional needs.

Assuming your goal is to maintain a healthy weight, it's probably in your best interest to focus on learning how these systems work in conjunction with one another and adopting a sustainable routine that keeps them, and therefore you, in balance.

FOODS TO CONSIDER

Now that we understand the basics behind two of the major nutritional pathways in your body and what you can do to keep them in balance, it's time to look at what types of food you may want to consider and in what proportions. This is a heavily nuanced topic that will depend on your specific preferences and goals, but there are some basic frameworks that most people can follow.

Before we dive into specific foods and macronutrients, I want to emphasize that this isn't about achieving nutritional perfection. The journey toward healthier eating isn't about getting everything right immediately or following every recommendation to the letter. It's about gradually building awareness and making incremental improvements where you can.

If the idea of calculating protein grams or tracking fiber intake feels overwhelming right now, that's completely normal. Full disclosure: I don't track my own calories or macros, I just use my knowledge of nutrition to make informed choices because I have a general idea of my required energy balance after doing this for long enough—for example, if I run a 10K I tend to eat more than on the days I'm less active. The information I'm sharing isn't meant to be prescriptive, but rather to empower you with knowledge that you can apply in ways that feel manageable and sustainable for you.

Some people might want to follow these guidelines more literally, while others may find themselves making more minor changes to their eating habits. Both approaches are absolutely fine. The important thing to remember is that even small, sustainable changes—like adding a salad to your dinner or choosing olive oil instead of saturated fats—can result in significant changes over time.

Another thing I'd like to clarify upfront is that while there are many different diet "camps" (keto, carnivore, vegan, paleo, and Mediterranean, etc.), when we look at what the *evidence* says, not all of them are created equal. Not to disparage anyone, but some are more like cults than evidence-based camps, although there are positive attributes of many of them. The reality is that there's little evidence to support that adhering to any one of these over another is best for your health in the long term. (I can feel the eyes glaring at me through the page.)

There is, however, plenty of evidence that supports adhering to a whole food, plant-based, minimally processed (ideally non-processed), and/or Mediterranean style diet. Healthy plant-based diets, which are higher in fiber, whole grains, vegetables, fruits, nuts, legumes, tea, coffee, fish, and lower in red meat, have been associated with a lower risk of cardiovascular disease mortality and all-cause mortality. There, I said it.

I am also aware that most if not all of the diets I just mentioned share many of these characteristics, but not all of them. The point is, if you want to feel and perform better, and ideally live longer, what you eat should follow an evidence-based framework and be tailored to your preference and individual considerations, which is why I wouldn't feel the need to stick to one specific diet camp.

> Ideally, you'll want to do your best to find locally sourced, fresh, organic products free from pesticides. And be sure to always wash your food before consuming!

That's a pretty broad realm of food to choose from. So, what specifically should you be focusing on within that umbrella? Well, it mostly comes down to getting the right proportions of macro and micronutrients. Eating a variety of fruits and vegetables will provide you with most of your required micronutrients, and the rest can be gained through supplementation—the focus of Chapter 9—so we'll skip those for now. The macronutrients, however, are worth understanding.

For those new to nutrition, there are three main macronutrients you consume in your food sources that your body can utilize for energy in one form or another; protein, fat, carbohydrates. Our focus here will mostly be on proteins, fats, and fiber (which is technically a type of carbohydrate).

PROTEIN

Many people associate protein with bodybuilding and putting on muscle, as if those are the only reasons to incorporate protein into your diet. While it is true that protein is required for muscle growth, it is incredibly relevant for everyone regardless of their activity level or fitness goals. Your body is quite literally made up of protein—about half the dry weight of your cells—so it only makes sense to prioritize protein in your diet. There is ample data supporting this.

One interesting feature of protein is related to something called the thermic effect of food, which is the amount of energy your body uses to digest, absorb, and metabolize the food you eat. Protein has the highest thermic effect of all macronutrients, meaning that for every gram you eat, your body actually burns about 30 percent of that just to process it. So, you're really only taking in closer to 70 percent of the protein-based calories you consume, which is one way protein can help you stay leaner.

This is quite different from fats and carbohydrates, where your body burns far fewer of those calories during digestion. Fats are incredibly energy-dense molecules that have over double the energy per gram of protein and carbohydrates, and only about a 5–10 percent thermic effect, meaning it is far easier for your body to store more calories when consuming fat. For carbohydrates, the energy per gram is about the same as protein; however, with a thermic effect of only 5–15 percent, they are still easier to over consume—not to mention people tend to enjoy them. This is one reason why the idea of "calories in, calories out" is an oversimplification. Different macronutrients have different metabolic impacts, although the principle of lowering caloric intake and increasing the relative amount of calories burned is more or less correct when it comes to maintaining a healthy lean mass or in planning a healthy pattern of weight loss.

The goal here should be to focus on consuming high-quality protein, ideally organically sourced, whether animal or plant-based. As we've covered, it may be helpful to know that plant-based proteins tend to activate mTOR less, whereas animal proteins and BCAAs (leucine, isoleucine, and valine) activate it more. Depending on your goals, it might make sense to prioritize one over the other.

The FDA currently recommends a protein intake of about 0.36 grams per pound of body weight per day, which probably means nothing to you if you aren't already keeping track of your macronutrients. That said, this target is likely too low to maintain a healthy lean mass for most people, not to mention prevent age-related muscle loss. 1.5 to 2.2g/kg/day, or 0.68 to 1g/lb/day of protein intake is likely more optimal for adequate muscle protein synthesis (although there is still some scientific debate here).

If this feels like a lot of math, don't worry—you probably don't need to get into decimals when calculating your own protein intake. The simple rule of thumb for anyone wanting to maintain lean muscle mass is to aim to eat close to your weight (in pounds) in grams of protein per day. For example, if you weigh 130 pounds, you would aim to consume approximately 130 grams of protein daily.

To be clear, this calculation should reflect your *lean mass* and not your additional adipose or fat mass. For example, if someone weighs 230 pounds, but 100 of those pounds consist of excess fat, they would still have the same goal of closer to 130 grams of protein per day since their lean mass is around 130 pounds.

Just to put some of these numbers into perspective, a typical chicken breast or one cup of chopped chicken has around 43 grams of protein. If you weigh 130 pounds, you would therefore need to consume around three chicken breasts worth of protein per day. If you weigh 180 pounds, that would be more like four chicken breasts. This might sound like a lot, and frankly, it is, which begs the question of how necessary this is. Again, there's still debate on whether this is truly the "correct" amount of protein to have in your diet, and the true amount appears to differ depending on which age group you fall in. However, the current evidence tells us that consuming sufficient protein to maintain strength and a healthy lean mass as you age appears to be the most correlated with improved longevity.

There is also conflicting data on exactly how much protein you can absorb per sitting, but it's thought to be around 50 grams per meal although this varies from person to person. More protein in one sitting is not known to be harmful; it's just not able to be utilized, and therefore, either not absorbed or converted and stored as fat. This would indicate that spreading your protein consumption across meals is ideal. Plus, you have the added bonus of not needing to eat four chicken breasts in one sitting. (Obviously, you don't need to eat chicken breasts despite what some fitness influencers might tell you. Any high-quality plant- or animal-based protein will do.)

HEALTHY FATS

Healthy fats are essential to your body, despite the bad reputation they received in the 1990s. That outdated belief that "fat is bad" unfortunately still lingers today, but it's mostly untrue. Case in point: your brain is approximately 60 percent fat. Adequate fat intake, therefore, is crucial for optimal brain health. Period.

Fats are defined generally as either **unsaturated** (liquid at room temperature) or **saturated** (solid at room temperature). Healthy fats primarily come from unsaturated sources like avocado, nuts, olive oil, wild fish like salmon, flaxseed, eggs, and natural cheese. While saturated fats are necessary in small doses, most people probably receive more than they need in their diets. Overexposure to saturated fats like those found in red meats, fried foods, and many other processed foods can be problematic—particularly because they can elevate your risk of cardiovascular disease, especially when paired with excess carbohydrates and refined sugar (this is currently another area of great debate, but sugar appears particularly problematic). As a general rule, most people would likely benefit from achieving about

20–35 percent of their total caloric intake from fat (most of which should be unsaturated), with no more than 10 percent of their total calories coming from saturated fat.

When it comes to healthy fats, fresh, organic, extra virgin olive oil is a personal favorite of mine and one that has been shown to have outsized benefits for your longevity. Olive oil contains a compound called **oleic acid,** which activates a family of longevity-related proteins called sirtuins. It also has a high polyphenol count, which we know serve as powerful antioxidants. As mentioned in Chapter 3, one study from *JAMA* demonstrated that consuming just seven grams of olive oil per day reduced the incidence of dementia by as much as 28 percent.

Sirtuins are a type of protein that are involved in many cellular processes including epigenetic regulation, DNA repair, regulation of your metabolism, and more.

Worth noting, it is best to consume high-quality "first cold press" organic olive oil, consume it while it's fresh, and avoid heating it to the point of smoking. Although a bottle might last for months, once you crack it open, the polyphenols begin to oxidize, especially when exposed to light. Therefore, to achieve the maximum benefits, it would be best to consume within a week or two of opening. I would avoid buying large containers but rather opt for smaller bottles (around 500mL) that you can get through more quickly, and that are ideally stored in darker glass bottles.

FIBER

Fiber, which is technically a type of indigestible carbohydrate, is an often-overlooked macronutrient that has been associated with a multitude of health benefits. I think most people are aware of how fiber affects bowel movements and digestive health, but that's really just scratching the surface of what it can do for your body.

The FDA currently recommends 25–30 grams of fiber daily; however, most people do not even achieve this and should likely be closer to 40–50 grams per day. Ideally, this should also be a combination of soluble and insoluble fiber. Just for clarity, **soluble fiber** dissolves in water, whereas **insoluble fiber** does not.

The way soluble fiber works is by combining with water to form a gel-like substance in your digestive tract. This can slow the absorption of carbohydrates which can help you maintain healthy blood glucose levels. It's also a powerful fuel for your gut microbiome.

If you recall, gut dysbiosis is a major hallmark of aging, and an easy way to avoid this is to keep the population of your gut microbiome in a healthy balance. Increasing your soluble fiber intake is perhaps one of the best ways to accomplish this, as this acts as a prebiotic that helps feed the right species of bacteria in your gut, such as lactobacillus and bifidobacterium. This provides a substrate (food source) for these bacteria to ferment into postbiotics like short-chain fatty acids and other signaling molecules that are essential to your health. This relationship was previously not well-understood, but it has become clear how necessary this is to keep you healthy and slow your body's rate of aging.

> **Prebiotics** are non-digestible food components that selectively stimulate the growth and/or activity of beneficial bacteria in the gastrointestinal tract. **Postbiotics** are substances produced by beneficial bacteria as they metabolize prebiotics.

Insoluble fiber, on the other hand, doesn't dissolve in water and passes through your digestive system largely intact. You can think of this almost like a broom sweeping through your digestive tract. Insoluble fiber is also what helps maintain regularity by preventing constipation and speeding up the passage of food through your digestive tract. I know that's not the nicest sentence to read, but given what I've seen in hospitals, there are plenty of people who could benefit from that bit of knowledge. It also helps prevent colon cancer, so that's a substantial bonus.

Most whole plant foods contain both types of fiber in varying amounts, which is why a diverse, plant-rich diet is the best way to ensure you're consuming enough of both.

One reason I'm such an advocate for fiber is because there has been an increasing amount of evidence linking fiber to lower all-cause mortality, along with a whole host of other benefits. According to a 2015 meta-analysis looking at almost one million people, for every 10 gram increase in fiber intake per day, all-cause mortality was lowered by an additional 10 percent. Comparing the top third of fiber consumers to the lowest third, there was about a 16 percent lower risk of all-cause mortality between the two groups—just by eating more fiber! This benefit does taper off at higher levels, so you can't simply eat 200 grams of fiber and live to be 400, but the evidence is clear that most of us need more fiber than we currently consume, and this is no surprise when we think about all its potential benefits.

In addition to everything we've mentioned above, elevated dietary fiber has also been shown to lower hemoglobin A1c (HbA1c) and fasting glucose in diabetics. It can also assist with improving insulin sensitivity, weight loss, and reducing inflammation, all of which helps regulate your nutrient sensing systems and avoid chronic inflammation—two key hallmarks of aging we discussed in Chapter 4.

Hemoglobin A1c is a measurement of your average blood sugar (glucose) levels over about the previous 3 months. More literally, it is the amount of sugar that is stuck to your red blood cells. (Crazy, right?)

A fiber-rich diet has also been shown to lower your risk of cardiovascular disease, particularly by lowering serum glucose and cholesterol levels and helping to normalize blood pressure. Promoting a healthy gut microbiome also improves your gut barrier, thereby reducing inflammation, improving your immune system function, and decreasing the risk of certain types of cancer such as colon and breast cancer, as we've also mentioned.

As if that weren't enough, high-fiber foods can also help you feel fuller for longer, which can help with decreasing your overall daily caloric intake and optimizing your weight management, resulting in a healthy ratio of lean to fat mass. Fiber is incredibly useful for your body and should be a core consideration of any proper nutrition plan. This is one reason I'm not a huge fan of diets like the Carnivore Diet, which may significantly reduce the intake of excess carbohydrates—which is a good thing—but by definition completely avoids fiber.

THINGS TO AVOID

The evidence shows us that protein, healthy fats, and fiber should be prioritized in most longevity-focused nutrition plans. Just as critical, however, is what should be avoided. Unfortunately, a significant portion of what you'll find in the middle aisles at your local grocery store should be avoided. Why? Because practically every processed food today has added sugar, preservatives, dyes, and additives that are not only nutritionally poor, but can cause a host of problems on their own.

For years, this problem has been exacerbated in the United States due to our lack of regulation around additives in food. I'm pleased and encouraged to see that the US is now starting to address this issue on a larger scale, by regulating the use of chemicals and preservatives that have been banned in other countries for decades. If you've had the opportunity to travel abroad and consume truly fresh food free of these, you'll understand the difference I'm talking about.

My goal with this section is not to make you feel guilty about what you eat or as if certain foods are "forbidden," but to help you understand what you're actually consuming, how it affects your body, and most critically, how that all aligns with your why. Growing up, I ate my fair share of processed foods, and I still do on rare occasions. I am by no means immune to the powers of the processed food industry. But now that I have a deeper understanding of what's in these products and how they may affect my body, I am inclined to avoid them because I know they don't serve me or my why. And speaking from experience, the hardest one for me to avoid is processed sugar.

PROCESSED SUGAR

Processed sugar is easily number one on the list of ingredients to avoid based on what we know. While molecular sugar, or glucose, is absolutely essential to your survival, how you get it in your diet matters. Your body is designed to obtain glucose from complex carbohydrates—like fruits, vegetables, and starches—that release it into your bloodstream slowly. Modern processed sugar, on the other hand, is like the equivalent of turning on a glucose firehose in your body.

Refined sugar bypasses your normal digestive mechanisms, causes an increased release of dopamine, and instantaneously activates the reward and addiction centers in your brain. These are literally the same regions that light up when people use substances such as cocaine and opiates. This can lead to a vicious addiction cycle that increases your cravings and a propensity to consume more sugar, which increases your risk of many of the chronic diseases we've covered.

The problem is that refined sugar is added to almost every processed food in the grocery store. You would be shocked at the number of products that contain added sugar—even savory foods that don't taste sweet have sugar listed in their ingredients. If you don't believe me, next time you're at the grocery store, pick up any packaged food in the middle aisles and you'll find that nearly all of them contain added sugar. Unfortunately, this is no accident. As mentioned in Chapter 1, the food industry knows that sugar can create a powerful addiction that keeps you coming back to buy more of their products.

Sugar-sweetened beverages are perhaps the worst offenders—sodas, fruit juices, sports drinks, sweet tea, etc. Multiple studies have linked their consumption with an increased risk of obesity and type 2 diabetes, with each additional drink furthering that risk. This of course makes sense, considering they provide virtually no sustenance yet are incredibly high in calories by way of refined carbohydrates. The same applies to sweets such as desserts and candy made almost entirely of processed sugar. Full disclosure—I struggle the most with the former, as I have a hard time saying no to dessert. We're in this together!

What helps me push additional sweets away, however, are the even more unsettling long-term effects sugar can have on other organs such as your brain and liver. There's a substantial link between increased processed sugar intake and accelerated cognitive decline, very likely due to many of the mechanisms we've discussed previously, which accelerate underlying cellular aging and advance the grip of chronic disease throughout your body.

Increased sugar consumption, particularly fructose, has been shown to cause a condition called non-alcoholic fatty liver disease, or NAFLD for short. This results in an excess buildup of fat in the liver, which can cause inflammation and liver dysfunction early on, but can progress to fulminant liver failure if left untreated—which is an organ you cannot live without. For context, if you were to look at the liver of someone with advanced NAFLD, it would look almost exactly the same as someone with liver cirrhosis from years of alcohol abuse.

Earlier in this chapter, we discussed the two main pathways affected by nutrition: AMPK and mTOR. If you recall, most people could likely benefit from an increase in AMPK activity and less mTOR. If you've been paying attention, you have likely already figured out that processed sugar does the exact opposite! By causing a massive insulin spike, processed sugar is a major activator of mTOR, which increases fat storage, decreases insulin sensitivity, and also makes it more difficult to lose weight, all while downregulating AMPK.

To really drive the point home, here are a few of the other ways processed sugar can result in chronic problems within your body.

- **Chronic inflammation:** Sugar consumption triggers inflammatory processes throughout your body, which we already know contributes to a variety of chronic diseases.
- **Cardiovascular risk:** Research has consistently linked high sugar intake with increased risk of coronary artery disease and heart complications.
- **Cancer:** Several types of cancer show higher rates of incidence in populations with elevated sugar consumption.
- **Visceral fat accumulation:** Sugar increases visceral fat in particular—the dangerous type of fat that surrounds your organs, which increases the production of inflammatory cytokines, and is strongly linked to metabolic diseases.
- **Blood glucose instability:** The rapid spikes and crashes from refined sugar consumption create a rollercoaster effect on your blood sugar levels. Research shows that maintaining steady glucose levels correlates with greater longevity by preserving insulin sensitivity and balancing metabolic pathways such as appropriate nutrient sensing.

With all that said, I wouldn't say that processed or refined sugar is "poison," despite catchy headlines you may read, but it should be avoided at nearly all costs. If possible, desserts that achieve their sweetness from natural substances like fruit or honey (ideally preceded by a heaping dose of fiber) are preferable to those with refined sugars—although they should still be consumed in moderation.

SOYBEAN OIL

As of writing this, there's been a lot of recent talk about seed oils being problematic. Big Seed Oil, anyone? The bottom line is that the data remain somewhat unclear and some appear better than others. The one to consider avoiding above all else is likely soybean oil. Like sugar, soybean oil is ubiquitous in processed foods. Once again, take a look next time you're at the grocery store—it is in a shocking amount of processed foods.

Perhaps the biggest problem with soybean oil is that it's very calorically dense, meaning it's easy to over-consume, which quickly results in an energy surplus for your body. The same could be said about nearly all cooking oils, yet soybean oil makes its way into foods that normally wouldn't even have oil in the first place—all because it's cheap and helps with the manufacturing process. That, plus all the added sugar, is one reason processed foods often contain significantly more calories than their homemade counterparts.

Soybean oil can also be used in many vegetable oil blends, so "vegetable oil" is worth carefully examining, as well. It's also worth noting that nearly all fast food establishments and many restaurants use vegetable oil to fry their foods—while I can't say for sure how much of that is soybean oil, it's safe to say that avoiding fried foods is generally a good idea.

Another trait that makes soybean oil particularly awful is that over 90 percent of it is genetically modified and often contains high levels of **glyphosate,** the chemical compound in Roundup weed killer. For reference, in 2015 the International Agency for Research on Cancer classified glyphosate as "probably carcinogenic to humans" meaning it likely causes cancer. There is also some evidence in animals that it can cause disruption to the endocrine system, which may also be the case for people. While the EPA (Environmental Protection Agency) did classify it as "practically nontoxic," I am personally skeptical of this stance. If you've ever sprayed a plant with Roundup, you'll know that nine times out of ten it is dead within 24 hours. So, I would ask yourself, "Am I willing to put this in my body?" I know my answer.

To "round out" this section (pun intended), soybean oil also contains high levels of omega-6 fatty acids, which have been associated with an increased risk of cardiovascular disease likely due to increased inflammation. These are very different from the anti-inflammatory omega-3 fatty acids found in fish oil, which do the opposite, and are a key supplement we'll be covering in Chapter 8. To be clear, there is some debate on whether excess omega-6s are in and of themselves harmful, or if the ratio of omega-6 to omega-3 is more relevant, but in either case an excess should likely be avoided.

Olive, avocado, pumpkin seed, grapeseed, and sesame oils all appear to be more or less okay when consumed in moderation. If using these to cook, be sure to keep them on low heat and do not let them smoke, as this can denature the oil and form trans fats, which are very unhealthy for blood vessels, not to mention aerosolized particles like aldehyde, which can be harmful if inhaled. For reference, the manufacturing of trans fats has actually been *banned* in the United States if that tells you anything, considering what we still allow. However, like all oils, you'll still want to be mindful of their overall intake as these are all similarly calorically dense.

INGREDIENTS YOU CAN'T PRONOUNCE

Another good rule of thumb is that if you can't pronounce or don't recognize an ingredient on the label, you probably shouldn't be eating it on a consistent basis. Many of these ingredients—which can be even more of a mouthful than some of the scientific jargon in this book—are synthetic preservatives, dyes, and additives that don't add any nutritional value to your food but may cause problems.

Given current evidence, we know that certain types of food dyes have been linked with increased cancer in animals. I certainly won't be surprised if further evidence comes out linking many of these ingredients to other problems, and recently this year the dye Red 3 was federally banned due to concerns over increased risk of cancer and possible hypersensitivity reactions. The reality is that most of these ingredients are relatively new, having been developed and added to our food supply within the last few decades, meaning it could still take some time to observe some of their long-term effects let alone understand all the mechanisms at play. Considering they have virtually no known benefits outside of preserving food we probably shouldn't be eating anyway, I would suggest avoiding them as much as possible.

In particular there is evidence supporting the avoidance of nitrates, potassium bromate, Red 3, Red 40, Yellow 5, and Yellow 6, PFAS, BHA, BPA, and heavy metals, among many other synthetic compounds.

MICROPLASTICS

Microplastics are another category that have also emerged as a new, invisible threat. And while I could have probably written an entire chapter on microplastics covering where they come from, how they're absorbed into our bodies, and the effects they have on our bodies, particularly the brain...I figured I'd spare you that tangent.

Without going into too many details, microplastics are ubiquitous in our environment. (As a side note, it's saddening to write about all these terrible things that are "ubiquitous," but that is unfortunately the world we live in.) Microplastics can cause a number of known problems, and we're learning more about them every year—most of which isn't great so far. Increased inflammation, disruption to the endocrine system, and dysbiosis are just a few areas of concern. More recently, microplastics have been found in increased quantities inside the brains of deceased people with dementia, and have also been found in arterial plaques, raising questions about their relationship to both conditions.

The good news is, you do have a large degree of control over limiting your exposure, and doing so is entirely possible through simple changes to your lifestyle and the products you have around your house. In general, here are some interventions to consider:

- Drinking out of glass bottles and cups, instead of plastic
- Filtering your drinking water with a reverse osmosis water filtration system
- Avoiding plastic cutting boards and Tupperware
- Avoiding the microwaving of plastic containers or drinking hot beverages out of paper or plastic containers (the former are lined with plastic, believe it or not)
- Avoiding the consumption of canned foods, which are also lined with microplastics
- Washing your food
- Eating organic foods if possible
- Exercise and regular sauna use, which may increase the rate of elimination of microplastics

FINAL CONSIDERATIONS FOR YOUR NUTRITION PLAN

Focusing on a whole food, organic, plant-based, minimally processed (ideally non-processed) nutrition plan is a great step toward living a longer, healthier life. Getting the right macronutrients, in the right proportions, while being mindful of your overall energy balance, is an even better step. This alone would put you far ahead of the vast majority of Americans in terms of your metabolic health and overall longevity.

However, there are a few more nuanced interventions to consider. While the above content should apply to most people, these last interventions are a bit more specific—they may or may not apply to you, based on your specific goals, preferences, and lifestyle. I would encourage you to experiment with what works best for you as you refine your nutrition plan.

With that said, here are some things worth considering:

- Eating your vegetables first (the order in which you eat your food matters)
- Avoiding snacking
- Intermittent fasting
- Wearing a continuous glucose monitor

Let's take a look at what the evidence says about each, so you can make an informed decision about how to proceed in your own life.

EAT YOUR VEGETABLES FIRST!

It turns out the order in which you eat your food matters. A calorie burned results in a fairly standard amount of energy expended, but a calorie consumed is not necessarily the same depending on the order in which it was consumed, its energy density, and the thermic effect of the given macronutrient.

Consuming soluble fiber allows the formation of that gel-like substance which coats the small intestine, promotes a healthy gut microbiome, and actually blocks and slows the absorption of some dietary sugar. Therefore, prioritizing fiber consumption first can circumvent some of the adverse effects we discussed previously, resulting in fewer carbohydrate-based calories absorbed—which, if you are trying to lose weight or even maintain a healthy weight like most people, is probably a good thing.

So, when you sit down for a meal, as strange as this may sound, a metabolically ideal order of consumption would be vegetables and fiber first, then protein and fat, and carbohydrates last. This can help regulate and maintain healthy blood glucose levels, and can even improve your metabolic health. Yes, this does mean the bread basket before dinner is probably not a great idea and that having a salad before your main meal would be a better option. Turns out mom was right when she told you to eat your vegetables.

Is this going to make or break your nutrition? Probably not. But it's an easy shift to make, one that can absolutely make a difference over time, and certainly worth considering.

AVOIDING SNACKING

We've already clarified that overeating is a problem because it keeps mTOR activated, putting you in a perpetual state of "building" and "storage" that leads to increased insulin resistance, weight gain, inflammation, and more. It also likely shortens your lifespan due to the inhibition of AMPK.

One of the easiest and most subtle ways to overeat is through snacking, especially when you consider that most "snack foods" are highly processed and calorically dense, with little nutritional value. Avoiding snacking, therefore, can be an effective strategy to curb overeating and reduce your overall calorie intake.

What's more, going for long periods of time without eating will activate AMPK, which we know is a good thing for longevity. I should clarify that you don't *have* to go for long stretches without eating to activate AMPK—maintaining a caloric deficit, meaning you are burning more calories than you consume, will still accomplish this regardless of how often you eat.

If you're struggling to lose weight or maintain a lean body mass, you may want to consider limiting your snacking in favor of eating more spaced out meals filled with whole foods and plant-based proteins.

INTERMITTENT FASTING

Unless you've been living under a rock, you've probably heard about the intermittent fasting craze. Over the last decade, intermittent fasting has worked its way into the popular lexicon as a way to lose weight and maintain a lean body mass.

Intermittent fasting is probably a healthy thing to do if your body can tolerate it. There's plenty of evidence showing that it does provide some immediate and long-term health benefits, which mostly comes down to the fact that it upregulates AMPK and downregulates mTOR. However, it's not a blanket strategy that can work for everyone.

Type 1 diabetics, for example, are dependent on insulin and must be very mindful of when they eat, so intermittent fasting can be dangerous for them. Some people also have a hard time fasting because of their daily routine. If you're a construction worker who's on the job site by 7:00 AM with a full day of grueling manual labor ahead of you, for example, skipping breakfast may not be the best idea. Assuming there is not a medical necessity to eat more often, and depending upon your personal goals (i.e., you're not a bodybuilder or already undernourished), consistently fasting for 12–16 hours within a 24-hour period is probably healthy from a metabolic perspective.

As far as how to specifically incorporate this into your lifestyle, there are many different types of fasting, all of which have been shown to help improve metabolic health:

- **ADF or alternate daily fasting:** alternating between normal eating days and days with very restricted or no calorie intake
- **The 5:2 method:** eating normally five days a week while restricting calories to about 500–600 per day on two non-consecutive days
- **TRF or time-restricted feeding:** limiting all food consumption to a specific window, typically eight to ten hours per day
- **IF or intermittent fasting:** a broader term encompassing various patterns of cycling between periods of eating and fasting
- **PF or periodic fasting:** longer fasting periods of 2–7 days done less frequently, such as monthly
- **Quarterly fasting:** extended fasting done four times per year, often aligned with seasonal changes

That said, the general guideline of fasting for 12–16 hours at a time is a good place to start if you're considering experimenting with this. Remember, you want a balance of autophagy, healthy cell turnover, and adequate muscle and protein synthesis. That happens when AMPK and mTOR are in balance, which you can achieve largely through nutrition—and *when* you eat plays a big role in this. We know that Alzheimer's, Parkinson's, and a host of other disorders result from an accumulation of intracellular protein inclusions, which are thought to stem from a defect in autophagy and are likely related to metabolic health.

The "fasting-mimicking diet" proposed by Dr. Valter Longo may also be worth considering for people with type 2 diabetes or metabolic syndrome. This is a five-day low-calorie, high-fat, low-protein, and low-carbohydrate diet which has been demonstrated to substantially improve insulin sensitivity, blood glucose levels, metabolic health, and HbA1c. For someone who is metabolically healthy, a fasting-mimicking diet once per quarter is likely sufficient if tolerable. If you're interested in learning more, I recommend his book, *The Longevity Diet*.

WEARING A CONTINUOUS GLUCOSE MONITOR

A continuous glucose monitor (CGM) can provide valuable insights into how your food choices affect your blood sugar in real time. It's worth noting that these can be expensive and are typically not covered by insurance unless you have diabetes. They are by no means necessary, but they can be helpful in the short term if you're looking to really refine your nutrition plan.

For the average person, this really only needs to be used for a month or two in order to obtain the data you need. Most CGMs link to an app on your smartphone and provide real-time data on your blood glucose levels. This can provide valuable feedback on your daily routine as you observe your body's response to different types of food intake. Over the course of a few months, you can start to understand how certain foods affect your blood glucose levels and how you can adjust your daily eating habits to maintain steady levels and avoid spikes, which has been correlated with increased longevity.

There are a handful of brands to consider, such as Dexcom, Medtronic, FreeStyle Libre, and Eversense, to name a few. They're all fairly similar, so I recommend doing your own research to determine which one will suit your needs best.

SHIFTING YOUR MINDSET

If there's one thing I want you to take away from this chapter, it's the simple mindset shift that *food is your body's fuel*. What you put into your body matters, and small changes to your nutrition plan over the long term can make a substantial difference in terms of your performance and longevity. While exercise is the biggest lever you have toward a longer, healthier life, nutrition comes in at a close second. It's also worth noting that exercise is far less impactful without a proper nutrition plan. In the fitness world, it's often said "you can't out-train a bad diet," which is largely true.

The key to long-term success with your nutrition is finding a sustainable approach that works for you, based on what we know the evidence says. Like with exercise, you can download the "nutrition cheat sheet" at TranscendHealthGroup.com/Resources which contains all the high-level information from this chapter, so you can hand-pick which interventions you'd like to incorporate into your own life. The key takeaway is that this should be sustainable and work for you in the long run. Allowing yourself the occasional dessert or piece of fried food is okay, as long as the vast majority of what you're consuming is the right food in the right amounts.

You truly are what you eat. The building blocks that make up your body are replaced continuously, and the quality of those replacements depends entirely on the nutrition you provide. *Every bite is an investment in your future self.*

KEY TAKEAWAYS

1. **AMPK and mTOR should be kept in balance.** Your nutrition plan directly affects these critical cellular pathways: AMPK (which promotes cellular cleanup, fat burning, and longevity) and mTOR (which builds muscle but can accelerate aging when overactivated). Overactivation of either is harmful, but most people will benefit from increasing AMPK activation through practices like time-restricted eating, while limiting mTOR activation by avoiding overeating or excessive animal proteins.

2. **Prioritize protein, healthy fats, and fiber in your diet.** These macronutrients form the foundation of any effective nutrition plan. Aim for 0.7–1g of protein per pound of body weight daily to maintain muscle mass, include healthy fats like olive oil for brain health, and consume 40–50g of fiber daily from plant sources to support gut health and lower all-cause mortality.

3. **Avoid processed foods, added sugar, and certain oils.** Processed sugar, soybean oil, and ingredients you can't pronounce contribute to inflammation, accelerated aging, and increased disease risk. Whole, minimally processed foods are a much better alternative. Strategies like eating vegetables first, avoiding late-night eating, and monitoring blood glucose can also be helpful.

You can find a list of all the specific interventions from this chapter in the Nutrition Cheat Sheet at TranscendHealthGroup.com/Resources.

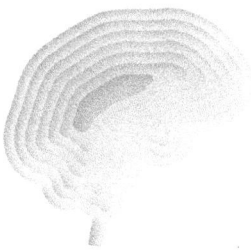

CHAPTER 7
SLEEP

THOMAS SAT ACROSS from me in my office, nervously fidgeting in his chair. At 45, he should have been in the prime of his life, but his weight and the dark circles under his eyes told a different story.

"Doctor Williamson, I've tried everything," he said, his voice heavy. "I'm eating better, I've joined a gym, but I can't lose this weight. And I'm just...exhausted. All the time."

Thomas had been referred to me for chronic, debilitating fatigue after his primary care physician had already run a thorough workup which revealed nothing out of the ordinary. On paper, he appeared relatively healthy. In person, he was anything but.

"I've reached the point where I'm falling asleep at my desk," he continued. "Last week, I nodded off at a red light. Just for a second, but it scared me."

His wife was seated beside him. When I asked about his sleep patterns, Thomas insisted he slept through the night—eight, sometimes nine hours.

"But it doesn't matter how long I sleep," he said. "I never feel rested."

I turned to Sarah. "Have you noticed anything unusual about his sleep?"

She hesitated, then nodded. "He snores—like a *chainsaw*. Sometimes..." she glanced at Thomas, "sometimes it seems like he has trouble breathing, too. Sometimes I lie awake listening to him, and suddenly there's this silence, and then he gasps for air. It terrifies me."

When I asked Thomas if he ever wakes up with headaches, his eyes widened. "How did you know? They're terrible! Every morning!"

It was clear to me that Thomas wasn't experiencing just fatigue. What I suspected, and what we soon came to discover, was that he had a condition called obstructive sleep apnea. So severe, in fact, that he stopped breathing on average *over 30 times per hour* during the night. In the absence of oxygen, his brainstem was constantly waking him up to try to keep air flowing into his lungs. This resulted in almost no meaningful or restful sleep, which led to multiple debilitating conditions including high blood pressure, insulin resistance, and his inability to lose weight—not to mention his fatigue, which was impairing his daily life.

Untreated sleep apnea is a ticking time bomb that significantly increases the risk of multiple life-threatening conditions, including heart attack and stroke. It can, therefore, be a silent killer. Fortunately for Thomas, a sleep study and subsequent treatment with a CPAP machine brought almost immediate relief. Within weeks, his energy began to return, his blood pressure normalized, and with proper sleep supporting his other health efforts, the weight finally began to come off.

SLEEP: THE LONGEVITY UNDERDOG

In my career as a neurologist, I've seen countless patients whose lives, like Thomas, have been dramatically altered by poor sleep. Whether it's the workaholic who says they'll "sleep when they're dead," or the patient with undiagnosed sleep apnea whose health is silently deteriorating, the reality is that sleep is not optional—it is essential.

Proper sleep is perhaps the best "bang for your buck" intervention in any longevity framework. Getting enough high-quality sleep has been shown to reduce your risk of dying from any cause and cut your chances of developing dementia by nearly 40 percent. It can significantly lower your risk of heart attack and stroke. It can improve your mood and simultaneously boost your cognitive performance and energy levels. Time and time again, studies have associated getting seven to nine hours of quality sleep per night with longer, healthier, and more disease-free lives. It also makes every day more enjoyable and productive, which helps you be more present for your mission in life and your why. You've surely experienced how great you feel after a good night's rest, and this is a very real, tangible daily goal.

The flip side of this equation is that a lack of sleep can be extremely problematic in both the short and long term—perhaps even more so than a lack of exercise or lack of proper nutrition. Regularly achieving less than seven hours of sleep over a twenty-four-hour period has been linked to a multitude of health problems from increased all-cause mortality to strokes, heart attacks, high blood pressure, metabolic syndrome, diabetes, obesity, increased cancer risk, seizures, depression, dementia, and so on.

Poor sleep can also negatively impact many of the other interventions we've discussed, leading to even more problems. If you're tired, you'll be less likely to exercise, for example. When you're tired you also tend to crave less healthy foods due to changes in your brain circuitry and hormones. To make matters even worse, you'll also probably lean more on caffeine to get through the day, which can negatively impact your sleep the following night. It's a vicious cycle and yet another example of how interrelated these mechanisms and interventions are.

Beyond the chronic health conditions, insufficient sleep immediately impacts your alertness, performance, judgment, memory, and ability to function throughout the day. To put this in perspective, staying awake for just seventeen hours—say, waking up at 7:00 a.m. and staying up until midnight—produces an impairment in your psychomotor skills equivalent to having a blood alcohol concentration of 0.05 percent. Extend that to twenty-four hours without sleep, and your level of impairment rises to the equivalent of a 0.1 percent blood alcohol level, well above the legal limit for driving in most states.

I experienced what a lack of sleep feels like firsthand during my medical residency, when twenty-four-hour calls were standard practice. Looking back, I can confidently say my decision making was substantially impaired relative to days when I was well-rested (which were still few and far between). This was not only unhealthy for me but potentially dangerous for my patients, yet remains a common practice in hospitals across the country.

Unfortunately, like so many of these chronic ailments, a lack of quality sleep is a common problem in our population. An estimated 50–70 million Americans suffer from insufficient sleep or at least one primary sleep disorder. That's roughly one in five people walking around every day with impaired cognition, increased risk of developing multiple chronic diseases, and shortened lifespans simply because they aren't achieving enough quality sleep.

So, why is sleep so crucial to your longevity, and what can you do to optimize it? Let's start by understanding what's actually happening when you close your eyes each night.

WHAT IS SLEEP?

Sleep is a complex, dynamic, and essential physiological state that is critical for maintaining your overall health and wellbeing. Despite taking up roughly a third of your life, sleep is not merely the absence of being awake—it's an *active* process dependent on multiple brain networks and is essential for sustaining life.

When you sleep, your body undergoes some interesting and measurable changes. Your heart rate and breathing slow down, your core body temperature lowers, your muscle tone decreases, and your brain waves cycle through distinct patterns as you progress through various sleep stages.

Perhaps even more fascinating is that all animals sleep in some form, which raises an interesting evolutionary question: why in the world would any species evolve to spend a third of its life in a vulnerable state, essentially defenseless against predators or natural disasters? The answer is that sleep serves such a fundamentally important role that it has been conserved across millions of years of evolution precisely because it too was essential to your ancestors' survival (hope they got that thank-you card)—and this has been consistently proven true as we've gained further understanding about how sleep affects our bodies and brains.

Ask any longevity expert from Peter Attia to Andrew Huberman, and they will all say that sleep is increasingly thought of as one of our biggest levers for increasing longevity. If you want to take a deep dive on the subject, I would highly recommend the book *Why We Sleep* by Matthew Walker, PhD, who outlines this fascinating subject better than anyone I've read.

This all certainly makes sense, when you consider the fact that sleep is the primary period when your body repairs and maintains itself and was essential to your development during childhood and adolescence. Sleep is a multifaceted state that impacts nearly every aspect of your body, *especially* your brain.

THE SCIENCE OF SLEEP

Sleep occurs in distinct stages, each of which serve specific purposes. These stages are defined by changes in your brain waves that can be measured with an electroencephalogram (EEG). There are four main stages: N1, N2, N3, and REM sleep. Although you'll often hear people group these into two broader stages:

1. Non-REM (NREM) sleep (N1, N2, and N3)
2. REM Sleep

When you first fall asleep, you enter light sleep (N1 and N2), followed by deep sleep (N3), and finally REM sleep. Throughout the night, you cycle through all these stages multiple times, with each complete cycle lasting approximately 90–110 minutes. The duration and order of these stages is referred to as your *sleep architecture*.

Interestingly, deep sleep occurs mostly during the first half of the night, while REM sleep is more prevalent toward the end. Deep sleep is where most of the repair and restoration happens, whereas REM sleep is where memories are consolidated. You also dream in REM sleep, which is why you often wake up in the middle of a dream—because you're more likely to be in REM sleep in the morning.

HOW YOU FALL ASLEEP AND WAKE UP

There are two main processes that initiate the onset of sleep: **Process S** and **Process C**. Both are important, and many of the subsequent interventions are designed to optimize these processes.

Process S: The Sleep Drive

Process S (sometimes called **sleep propensity** or the **homeostatic drive**) is essentially the mechanism that makes you feel sleepy. It is driven by the accumulation of the neurotransmitter adenosine, which gradually rises throughout the day, making you feel progressively more tired as the day goes on. This phenomenon is also known as **sleep pressure.**

At a cellular level, the way this works is that adenosine binds to various receptors across of your brain including many of the areas we covered in Chapter 2, like your cortex, hippocampus, thalamus, and basal ganglia. When adenosine binds to these receptors, it inhibits the networks that keep you awake and alert. Adenosine also induces sleep through its action on your thalamus, which is the walnut-sized relay center in the middle of your brain we discussed when we looked at motor control earlier.

The most important thing to understand is that you feel tired because of the accumulation of adenosine throughout the day. Interventions that limit the action of adenosine may help you feel more alert, but they may make it more difficult to fall asleep later.

Process C: The Body Clock

Process C is something you've likely heard of—the circadian alerting signal, also known as your **circadian rhythm.** This is your body's internal clock that regulates your level of alertness and sleep relative to light and dark cycles in your environment.

This process is driven by the daytime solar activation of the **melanopsin system** in your retinae, which line the backs of your eyes. Melanopsin is a light-sensitive pigment present within specialized neurons called retinal ganglion cells. When activated by solar light, these neurons send signals to multiple areas of your brain, including the **suprachiasmatic nucleus (SCN)** in the hypothalamus. The SCN is often described as the circadian pacemaker, synchronizing many of your bodily functions to the twenty-four-hour day-night cycle.

To grossly oversimplify this process, when your eyes detect incoming light, specialized neurons in your retinae send a signal to your brain that you should be awake. Furthermore, these same neurons send a signal to a tiny region of your brain just behind your thalamus called the **habenula**, which is thought to help regulate mood. This is partly why regular exposure to natural light, particularly early in the day, can have a largely positive impact on your overall mood.

One crucial aspect of your circadian system is its regulation of **melatonin**, a hormone that helps your brain initiate the onset of sleep. This happens largely thanks to your **pineal gland**, which is a tiny pea-sized gland that sits just behind your thalamus whose main function is to receive and convey information about the current light-dark cycle of your environment. In darkness, your pineal gland secretes melatonin, which signals to your body that it's time to sleep. Exposure to light, however—especially shorter wavelengths in the blue and green range—suppresses melatonin production, which can lead to you staying up well past your intended bedtime.

This can be a serious hindrance if you stare at screens late into the night, which as you know has become commonplace. This is also why there is so much talk around limiting screen time before bed. Most screens emit large amounts of blue frequency light waves, which suppresses the release of melatonin from your pineal gland. By looking at a screen late at night, you're essentially telling your brain that it's daytime and you should be awake. I'm sure you can understand why that's not great for your sleep.

This is another situation where human evolution has not yet caught up to technology. Before screens and even electricity were invented, this system served us very well. Now, it can cause problems. (Or, I suppose, screens are causing the problems—our brains are working exactly as intended!)

To recap, **Process S** refers to the buildup of a neurotransmitter (adenosine) that makes you feel progressively more tired throughout the day, and **Process C** is the system that tells your brain when to wake up and when to go to sleep relative to light exposure. Many of the interventions we will discuss are centered around balancing these two processes—so your daily routine works with them, not against them.

HOW SLEEP TRANSFORMS YOUR BODY AND BRAIN

We've already discussed how sleep impacts neural processes like memory retention, but it regulates many other critical functions, as well. At a high level, sleep helps you grow and develop, regulates your metabolism, clears waste products from your brain, consolidates memories, regulates your emotions, helps you recover from injury, maintains your immune system, improves your cardiovascular health, and preserves your cognitive function. In other words, it helps with nearly *all* the primary threats and hallmarks of aging we've discussed previously.

But this is really just scratching the surface. When you dig deeper into the science of sleep and how it affects various parts of your body, it becomes abundantly clear why this is such an important part of our lives. Given the knowledge you already have of your body and brain, it's worth spending some time on this to understand how sleep impacts many of the cellular mechanisms we've previously discussed.

Growth and Development

Sleep is the primary time you grow during your initial development. While some growth happens during the day, the majority of growth hormone (which tells your body to do exactly that) is released at night while you're asleep. This is one of the many reasons proper sleep is particularly crucial during childhood and adolescence.

This does not mean it's irrelevant to developed adults, as this is the primary time when muscle and tissue repair occurs throughout your body, in particular after vigorous exercise. Ask any bodybuilder and they'll tell you that sleep is just as important as protein intake when it comes to building muscle.

Metabolic Regulation

Impaired sleep can result in elevated fasting glucose, increased insulin resistance, and a higher risk of developing diabetes. Poor sleep also disrupts your hunger and satiety hormones, increasing a hormone called **ghrelin**, which makes you feel hungry (think of growling like you're "hangry"), and decreasing another hormone called **leptin**, which makes you feel full.

This hormonal imbalance can lead to overconsumption of calories simply because your brain signals to you that you're hungry when in fact your body doesn't require any further nutrition to sustain itself. Achieving proper sleep, on the other hand, can counteract this and can help regulate your metabolism.

Waste Clearance

Sleep is the primary time you clear waste products from your brain through your glymphatic system. This includes those previously mentioned proteins like amyloid-beta and tau (implicated in Alzheimer's disease), as well as alpha-synuclein (implicated in Parkinson's disease). For context, when you're awake, the flow of cerebrospinal fluid through this system decreases by as much as 60–90 percent, which substantially reduces your brain's ability to clear toxic waste products and misfolded proteins.

Disruption of this pathway can result in a vicious cycle. As these proteins accumulate, they further disrupt normal cellular functions, including the sleep-wake cycle, making it even more difficult to achieve adequate sleep, which in turn allows more abnormal proteins to accumulate. Over time, this can dramatically increase the risk of developing neurodegenerative disease.

Memory Consolidation

Sleep is the only time you consolidate newly formed memories (unless, of course, you haven't been sleeping well!). As we covered in Chapter 2, during sleep your short-term memories (which are temporarily held in your hippocampus) become converted to long-term memories in various regions of your brain where you can access them later for use.

If you aren't achieving an adequate volume of quality sleep on a consistent basis, you're essentially impairing the ability to register memories from parts of your life. I don't know about you, but I'd like to keep as many memories as possible, for as long as possible.

Emotional Regulation

We all know how irritable we can feel after a poor night's sleep—this isn't just a subjective experience, there are neurological and biochemical underpinnings as to why this happens. Sleep has been shown to help regulate emotions and cognition. Getting enough quality sleep not only benefits you, it likely benefits the people around you too! No one likes a grouch like Oscar.

Recovery and Healing
Sleep is largely for when you recover from exercise, physical activity, and injury. Interestingly, it also improves your pain tolerance and can even decrease the likelihood of headaches such as migraines in susceptible individuals.

Even if you don't have any specific injuries or ailments, your body is constantly maintaining all the routinely used machinery inside of you, and a large part of that takes place during sleep. If you think back to our general thesis of slowing down the rate of your cellular aging, sleep is one of the primary ways you can accomplish this by maintaining the function of your cells and the various systems of which they are a part.

Immune Function
Sleep is also necessary for the normal activation and functioning of your immune system. Improper sleep has been shown to decrease the activity of your natural killer cells by as much as 30 percent. These are the cells that help fight infection and kill cancer cells as they form. Poor sleep has been linked with an increased risk of several cancers, including breast and colon cancer. This is also why proper sleep is so beneficial when fighting off an infection.

Cardiovascular Health
Inadequate sleep can increase your risk of suffering a stroke or developing heart disease through multiple mechanisms. It can increase neuroinflammation and oxidative stress, contribute to increased mitochondrial damage, and the formation of a prothrombotic

state—all of which are key hallmarks of aging. Chronic sleep deprivation can also result in an increased resting heart rate, blood pressure, and activation of your sympathetic nervous system, which can impair the normal relaxation of your blood vessels, further elevating the risk of cardiovascular disease.

Poor sleep can also activate your immune system in ways that contribute to increased cholesterol formation and atherosclerosis (plaque buildup in your arteries), increasing the risk of heart attack and stroke. In short, if you're looking to optimize your cardiovascular health, quality sleep is an essential part of the equation.

Like exercise and nutrition, it has become increasingly clear that sleep is a non-negotiable for optimal longevity—and given this list of benefits, it's easy to see why. If you want to live a longer, healthier life and give yourself the best chance at achieving your why, achieving regular, high-quality sleep is absolutely essential.

And as with some of our other interventions, many of the problems we experience around sleep are not necessarily our fault, but the result of our modern lifestyle. Staring at a screen all day, stressing over deadlines at work, consuming caffeine to keep you going, having a few drinks to wind down—these are all easy habits to fall into, yet they counteract your body's natural sleep cycle. The good news, however, is that there are many simple, low-cost, evidence-based interventions you can implement to get back to a more natural sleep cycle. It's time to address those.

EVIDENCE-BASED INTERVENTIONS FOR BETTER SLEEP

As we begin to explore some of the evidence-based interventions for better sleep, it's worth keeping in mind that implementing all of these or achieving "perfect" sleep on a consistent basis may be a bit unrealistic for the average person, at least to start. There are, however, many small changes you can make to steadily improve your sleep over time. The goal is to use this information to craft a routine that works for you.

As much as I love sleep, I still sometimes find myself scrolling on my phone late at night when I know I shouldn't be or missing early light exposure when I have a busy day. That said, I don't obsess over it because I know that over the long term I am achieving enough high-quality sleep on most nights.
Whatever you can do to improve your sleep habits is a win, and there's no sense in beating yourself up about getting this perfect. In fact, that added stress would probably hinder your sleep!
So, without further ado, let's get into it.

FINDING YOUR CHRONOTYPE

We all have a chronotype, or a natural tendency to fall asleep and awake at certain times. Genetically, about one-third of us are early risers (often called "larks"), one-third are night owls, and the remaining third fall somewhere in between.

Your chronotype isn't just a preference—it's hardwired into your biology, affecting not just your sleep but your digestive processes, timing of hormone release, and cognitive performance throughout the day. All these systems are like a giant symphony that in many ways is directed by your chronotype, although it's worth noting your lifestyle can have a significant impact on all of this, as well.

Honoring your natural chronotype is a much better strategy than trying to fight against it, although many of the interventions below can help you work around it. That said, this can be challenging depending on your schedule—especially for night owls. If you want to give your boss a copy of this book to explain why you need to come in to work an hour late every day, you're welcome to do that. I can't say for sure how that will go, but you can certainly try and have my full support.

Most people have a decent sense of where their chronotype lies. If you're unsure, pay attention to when you naturally feel most alert and when you start to feel tired when you're on vacation or have several days free from scheduling constraints. This will give you a good indication of your natural rhythm.

CONSISTENCY

At this point, I've spoken at length about how consistency is beneficial for exercise and nutrition—but sleep is particularly unique in this regard. There is actually data showing that people who maintain consistent sleep schedules, *even if they're getting slightly less than the ideal amount of sleep,* often have better health outcomes than people who get adequate sleep on average but with significant day-to-day variability. The goal here is to try to maintain a consistent sleep and wake time. One simple strategy is to always aim to go to bed and wake up within an hour of what you did the previous day. For example, if you went to bed at 10:00 p.m. yesterday, don't stay up past 11:00 p.m. tonight.

And yes, this does apply on the weekends. If you have a great sleep schedule during the week but stay out until the wee hours of the night every weekend, you're really not doing yourself any favors. I wish I could go back and tell my college self this advice, although I don't think that guy would've been terribly receptive given his priorities at the time.

EARLY LIGHT EXPOSURE

Given what we now know about Process C, it should be no surprise that early morning light exposure is helpful for consistent sleep. Regularly practicing this habit helps to maintain your circadian rhythm and is almost like resetting your biological clock every morning to make sure it's as accurate as possible. This is also important because your natural circadian rhythm is actually slightly longer than twenty-four hours, which can lead to unintentionally staying up later and sleeping later over time if you do not continually provide this stimulus to train it. It also means you'll feel more awake and energized for your day, which is a massive performance enhancer.

According to current evidence, the best strategy is to get somewhere between 10–15 minutes of long wavelength light (ideally direct sunlight) every morning, or as often as you are able. Critically, if we're talking about sunlight, this should be when the light is still at a low angle and emitting red or orange colors—not bright light, as this can damage your eyes. This early in the day, however, you don't need to wear sunglasses, and in fact this can minimize its effectiveness, as can UV-filtering windows or glass.

So just enjoy being outside for a few minutes, face the sun or your preferred light source, and be sure to get the light in your eyes without staring directly at it. This could be during a walk or while sitting at home having your morning coffee. Not only does it help maintain your circadian rhythm, but it's also been shown to help improve your mood. Personally, my wife and I get early light exposure most mornings while walking our two dogs, and I've noticed an improvement in my sleep and mood—plus, it's a great way to start the day with intentional movement and to spend time together, which lowers stress and releases oxytocin, the safety hormone we covered in Chapter 2.

If you wake up later in the day (I'm talking to you, night owls), there are a variety of phototherapy lamps that can also help with this.

EXERCISE TIMING

Physical activity significantly impacts your sleep quality. Generally speaking, if you exercise during the day, you'll tend to sleep better at night—and this is particularly true with any type of intense training. However, the timing of exercise does make a difference. You can probably imagine how difficult it can be to go to sleep immediately after a hard workout. That's because exercise can increase your core body temperature, elevate your heart rate, and stimulate the release of hormones like adrenaline and cortisol—all of which can interfere with sleep onset if they occur too close to bedtime. In fact, a recent study in *Nature* looking at a year's worth of sleep patterns in over 14,000 people showed that exercise within four hours of bedtime, and particularly intense exercise, was associated with delayed sleep onset, shorter sleep duration, and lower sleep quality, which is perhaps no surprise.

Therefore, the ideal window for exercise is likely sometime in the morning or early afternoon, allowing your body ample time to naturally wind down before bedtime. That said, ideal timing depends somewhat on your chronotype. Early risers may perform better with morning sessions, while night owls may find the afternoon to be more effective. And in my opinion, any exercise is probably still better than exercise at the wrong time.

CAFFEINE INTAKE

Caffeine directly interferes with Process S—the buildup of sleep pressure—by blocking adenosine receptors. When caffeine occupies these receptors, adenosine can no longer bind to them, which means you don't feel the natural sleepiness that would otherwise eventually accumulate later in the day.

What many people don't realize is how long caffeine remains active in the body. The half-life of caffeine is approximately five to six hours for most people (although this varies), meaning that it takes five to six hours to deplete *by half.* That means half of the caffeine from your 2:00 p.m. coffee is likely still circulating in your bloodstream at 8:00 p.m. Complete clearance can take up to ten hours. This also means that the quantity of caffeine consumed does impact how long it stays in your body. Taking a large dose of caffeine early in the morning can still affect your sleep, potentially even more so than drinking small amounts later in the day.

Additionally, there's significant genetic variation in how we all metabolize caffeine. Some people are fast metabolizers who can drink coffee later in the day and fall asleep without issue, while others are slow metabolizers who might have sleep disruption from a morning cup or two. Anecdotally, I've met plenty of people who say caffeine doesn't affect them, which is probably more a reflection of overconsumption and tolerance than anything. Technically speaking, that's not really possible; caffeine absolutely affects everyone, some people are just more or less sensitive to it than others.

Regardless, even if you feel like caffeine doesn't affect you or you don't think it's impacting your sleep, it is generally a good rule of thumb to keep your intake moderate (not to the point you feel jittery and have heart palpitations) and limit consumption after noon. It's also worth noting that moderate caffeine consumption has been associated with some health benefits, including potential neuroprotective effects against conditions like Parkinson's and Alzheimer's. And while caffeine is most commonly associated with coffee, it is also found in many types of tea, chocolate, sodas, and some medications, although I'd recommend skipping the sodas for obvious reasons.

MEAL TIMING

Eating too close to bedtime can also disrupt sleep in several ways. When you consume food, your gut becomes activated and your brain receives signals that can interfere with your sleep-wake cycle, making it difficult to fall asleep and sleep well throughout the night.

There's also a fascinating relationship between your circadian rhythm and your metabolism. Your circadian pacemaker can actually be altered by feeding patterns, a concept researchers call **chrononutrition**. Eating too late can trigger increased production of cholesterol and potentially elevate cancer risk by deregulating genes related to suppressing cancer formation.

Given what we know about AMPK and mTOR, we also know that calories consumed later in the evening are more likely to be stored as fat rather than burned for energy as most people are likely more insulin-resistant later in the day. This is actually a technique that sumo wrestlers use to gain weight by eating high-carbohydrate meals before napping. So, if you're an aspiring sumo wrestler, I suppose you can avoid this advice—but I'm assuming most people aren't interested in developing that particular body habitus.

All jokes aside, avoiding late-night eating is also a great way to start working fasting into your routine if that's something you want to experiment with. For example, if you finish dinner by 6:00 p.m. and don't consume any calories after that, a twelve-hour fast would mean you could eat again at 6:00 a.m. A sixteen-hour fast would equate to 10:00 a.m. This is very doable for many, myself included. In my case, freshly ground black coffee and exercise in between helps keep my appetite suppressed.

ALCOHOL

Although alcohol may help you fall asleep initially it significantly impairs your overall sleep quality. That's because its **metabolites** (what's left in your bloodstream after it passes through your liver) remain in your bloodstream for three to four hours after your last drink, and continue to alter your sleep architecture throughout the night.

One of the many problems with alcohol is that it suppresses REM sleep during the first half of the night. As alcohol is metabolized, it can trigger a rebound effect with more frequent awakenings and sometimes vivid or disturbing dreams during the second half of the night.

Beyond sleep architecture, alcohol also impairs your body's temperature regulation and reduces heart rate variability (HRV), which can lead to unrestful sleep and contribute to other long-term health problems whether it is regularly consumed before bed or not. Even one drink per day has been associated with thinning of the cerebral cortex and resultant brain atrophy, accelerated loss of neurons, and loss of white matter integrity in large populations studied. I also unfortunately regularly encounter heavy drinkers in my clinical practice who suffer from irreversible dementia, neuropathies, and other chronic medical problems. That said, if you choose to drink, allowing at least three to four hours between your last drink and bedtime can help alleviate these effects on your sleep, and this is assuming you haven't oversaturated your body's capacity to process alcohol, which equates to about one drink per hour.

Alcohol consumption in general does not appear to be conducive to a healthy lifestyle, and to date there is no amount of alcohol that appears medically beneficial in any way—which *does* include red wine. The supposed benefits of red wine are often attributed to a compound called resveratrol, which does have some antioxidant properties. However, to receive any meaningful benefit from resveratrol via red wine, you would need to consume literally hundreds of glasses of wine in a day, which would obviously cause far more significant problems (like your immediate death, so please don't try this).

There is also a correlation between red wine consumption and longevity in certain populations, like Blue Zone residents, but my perspective is that these are likely explained by factors other than the wine itself. This has become a timeless and comical debate between my good friend and Certified Sommelier, Mario, who is convinced otherwise.

In my opinion, from an exclusively medical perspective, alcohol should likely be avoided at all costs. So it's clear I'm not throwing stones in a glass house and for the sake of full disclosure, I do personally enjoy a high-quality German beer or glass of wine with dinner *occasionally*, but I do my absolute best to keep it to a minimum. The improvements in my sleep, mood, stress response, and mental clarity have been overwhelmingly worth it.

ARTIFICIAL LIGHT EXPOSURE

Your ancestors lived in a world where sunset meant darkness and the end of their daily activities. Today, we're surrounded by artificial light at nearly all times of the day and night, which our circadian rhythm was simply not designed for.

As we discussed earlier, light exposure—particularly blue and green wavelength light—suppresses melatonin production. The light from your smartphone, tablet, computer, and TV is full of these shorter wavelengths, making screen use before bed one of the most common disruptors of healthy sleep. Studies show that even brief exposure to blue light in the evening can delay melatonin release *by up to three hours* and reduce the total duration of REM sleep. That means even if you can fall asleep quickly after looking at your phone, your overall sleep quality may still be affected.

Therefore, avoiding all screens for at least an hour before bedtime (if not longer) is an effective way to combat this issue, which I know can be challenging. If you must use screens in the evening, consider wearing blue light blocking glasses, which filter out the most disruptive wavelengths. Or ideally, instead of electronic devices, try reading a physical book under low, warmer (incandescent) lighting, which contains less blue light and is less disruptive to your melatonin production. Plus, reading is great for your brain! As a last resort, I know some great textbooks that are an instant cure for insomnia.

STRESS

As we've covered, chronic stress is harmful to your body in many ways, but when it comes to sleep it's particularly problematic because it keeps your sympathetic nervous system activated. As you may recall, this is your "flight or fight mode," in which your body increases the release of hormones like cortisol and adrenaline that increase your alertness, elevate your heart rate, and prepare you for action. It should go without saying that this is fundamentally incompatible with sleep. Your body needs to be in a relaxed state to fall asleep, and stress does the opposite.

Beyond those immediate effects, even low levels of chronic stress can lead to racing thoughts, worrying, and rumination that can make it difficult to fall asleep. If you've ever experienced this, it's incredibly frustrating—your racing mind keeps you awake long after you've gone to bed, only for you to become even more stressed because you're not sleeping. Not a great situation.

This is a challenging problem to solve, especially since most people can't just wave a magic wand and remove all sources of stress from their life, as lovely as that might sound. One helpful strategy can be to create a deliberate wind-down routine beginning at least one hour before bed. Turning the lights down, and activities like journaling, mindfulness meditation, sauna bathing (more below), or reading a physical book can be helpful here. Creating a list of tasks for the next day has also been shown to be helpful as it can clear your mind of lingering thoughts and prevent you from worrying about what needs to get done. Find what works for you, but be intentional about putting this into practice.

TEMPERATURE

Your core body temperature naturally begins to lower in the evenings prior to the onset of sleep in conjunction with your circadian rhythm, and sleeping in a slightly cooler environment has been shown to be helpful in assisting with this process.

Research shows that the ideal temperature for sleep is somewhere between 60–65°F (15.5–18.3°C), though your specific preference may vary. Sleeping in a warm environment can often disrupt sleep architecture—if you've ever spent a night in a hot bedroom without air conditioning, you can probably relate.

Lowering the temperature indoors around one to two hours before bedtime can help initiate this process. Interestingly, taking a *hot* shower or spending time in a sauna thirty minutes to an hour before bed can be helpful, as well. It's counterintuitive, but being in a warm environment like this actually lowers your core body temperature. In response to the ambient heat, the blood vessels in your skin dilate to help dissipate more heat, and your core temperature lowers as a result. When you then exit to a cooler indoor environment, this can help you maintain sleep as mentioned above.

This also means the opposite is true. Taking a cold plunge or cold shower causes your peripheral blood vessels to constrict and as a result your core body temperature actually rises. This also results in activation of your sympathetic nervous system via the release of more activating neurotransmitters. Therefore, I wouldn't recommend taking a cold plunge before bed. (We'll also discuss cold plunges in Chapter 8.)

DARK AND QUIET

Even minimal light exposure during sleep can disrupt your circadian rhythm and sleep quality. Light can actually penetrate your eyelids and signal to your brain that it's daytime, suppressing melatonin production and potentially causing you to shift between sleep stages inappropriately or even you wake up entirely.

Similarly, noise disruptions—even those that don't *fully* wake you—can cause enough of a stimulus to shift your sleep to lighter stages, reducing overall sleep quality. Believe it or not, your brain continues to process sounds during sleep, with certain areas remaining vigilant for potential threats or important signals. This provided another evolutionary advantage that helped keep your ancestors safe from predators, and certainly still has some use today—but you don't want to engage it unnecessarily.

Using an eye mask or blackout curtains are simple interventions that can help with this. Even small sources of light from LEDs on electronics can be disruptive, so it's best to cover those or simply turn them off if possible. Using earplugs or a white noise machine to block disruptive sounds can also be helpful.

MELATONIN

If you follow even a portion of the previously mentioned interventions, you should already be well on your way to better sleep. However, if you still find yourself struggling to fall asleep or perhaps you travel often and need help with jet lag, over-the-counter melatonin can be helpful.

As we've discussed, melatonin is your body's natural sleep hormone. The pills you can buy at the store are a manufactured version of the same thing, you're just getting an extra boost from a pill instead of relying solely on your pineal gland. Given our knowledge of the role melatonin plays in your circadian rhythm, supplements are particularly helpful for resetting your biological clock much like morning light does—and can be useful in recovering from jet lag or after periods of disrupted sleep.

Three to five milligrams fifteen to thirty minutes before bedtime can be helpful in these situations. Crucially, you'll want to be sure to keep your sleep environment dark when taking melatonin as light blocks its effectiveness. Melatonin also shouldn't be taken long-term (ideally no more than a month or two consistently) as it can downregulate your body's natural production of melatonin over time, which can lead to other problems.

While we're on the topic of sleep aids, I highly recommend avoiding benzodiazepines (Ambien, Lunesta, Belsomra, and the like) if you are able. These medications bind to the same receptors as alcohol, and while they may help you fall asleep, they too can significantly impair sleep architecture. This can result in non-restorative sleep and potentially harmful long-term effects to your health. If you've ever taken one of these and felt groggy the next morning, that can be due to circulating metabolites of these molecules or because your sleep likely wasn't as restorative as it should have been.

WEARABLES

There are a handful of wearable devices that can be very helpful in tracking your sleep patterns. Devices such as the Oura Ring, Apple Watch, or Whoop band all have these capabilities. These devices aren't perfect, but they can provide some valuable insights into your sleep patterns and how they change based on your behaviors and environment—kind of like how a continuous glucose monitor can show you how certain foods affect your blood glucose levels.

These should be viewed as tools to modify healthy sleep habits, rather than an absolute indicator of sleep quality. More on these in Chapter 10.

FURTHER ACTION

Consistent implementation of these interventions over the course of one to two months should provide significant improvement for most people. If you're following sound sleep habits and you're still not seeing an improvement in the quality or duration of your sleep, it may be time to consider whether or not you have an underlying sleep disorder.

Sleep orders can be diagnosed by a sleep specialist, who will likely conduct a study called a polysomnogram. This type of sleep study provides significantly more information than something like an at-home wearable device and can be used to diagnose conditions like sleep apnea, narcolepsy, and other primary sleep disorders.

For what its worth, obstructive sleep apnea is the most common sleep disorder, affecting an estimated 30 million adults in the United States, which is why I've encountered many patients like Thomas in my career. Sleep apnea is typically treated with a CPAP machine, which is incredibly effective at improving sleep quality for those affected, although there are other medical procedures and devices available too.

I feel I should point out that the CPAP machine you may be familiar with—the big mask that goes over the nose and mouth with a hose connecting to a bulky machine—has become a thing of the past. Newer CPAP machines are much more minimal, with some being as simple as a small breathing tube that connects to your nostrils. So, if you suspect you have sleep apnea but the idea of wearing one of those big masks is just too much for you, it might be time to look into this again, as it is a highly treatable condition that can lower your risk of chronic disease and potentially add years to your life.

SLEEP IS A CORNERSTONE OF HEALTH

Given my background in neurology, I've always found sleep particularly fascinating. It is an essential part of our lives that serves us in many ways—from brain health to recovery to lowering inflammation, and so much more. Sleep is almost like our own internal medicine, and it should absolutely be prioritized and treated as a non-negotiable.

I'm happy to see that in recent years, the longevity community has embraced this idea. Sleep is now being seen for what it is—an essential part of your physiology that when optimized can help you live a longer, healthier life. I therefore consider sleep optimization to be one of the most powerful interventions we have for improving daily cognitive performance, long-term brain health, and maintaining your body's critical functions. Adhering to a proper sleep, nutrition, and exercise routine will get you *very* far in life. Plus, it will make your day-to-day life much more enjoyable.

Remember that consistency is key. Getting a good night's sleep isn't going to change your life overnight (although it might change the next day), but it is another investment in your health. The more positive choices you make over time, the higher your return will be.

KEY TAKEAWAYS

1. **Sleep is a non-negotiable pillar of longevity.** Getting seven to eight hours of quality sleep nightly reduces all-cause mortality by up to 40 percent and cuts dementia risk by nearly 40 percent. Sleep deprivation negatively impacts everything from cognitive function to cardiovascular health and your immune response, making proper sleep just as essential as exercise and nutrition for extending your healthspan and lifespan.

2. **Sleep quality depends on two key processes:** Process S (sleep pressure from adenosine buildup) and Process C (your circadian rhythm) regulate when you feel sleepy and alert. Many of the sleep interventions we've discussed are centered around optimizing those two key processes, like maintaining consistent sleep-wake times, morning light exposure, timing exercise appropriately, and managing caffeine intake.

3. **Improve your sleep by optimizing your environment and routine.** The most effective sleep interventions include honoring your chronotype, maintaining consistent sleep-wake times (even on weekends), ensuring your bedroom is dark and cool (60–65°F), avoiding screens and large meals before bed, and creating a deliberate wind-down routine. These environmental factors can dramatically improve the quantity and, critically, the quality of your sleep.

You can find a list of all the specific interventions from this chapter in the Sleep Cheat Sheet at TranscendHealthGroup.com/Resources.

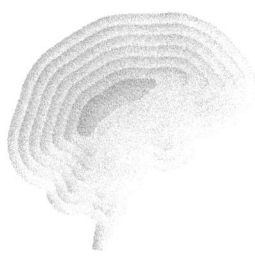

CHAPTER 8
HORMESIS AND STRESS MANAGEMENT

I WILL NEVER FORGET the first time I took a cold shower. Having read about the benefits of cold plunges and intentional cold exposure, I decided to finally give it a try one day. I had been in cold water before, so I thought, "This will be fun, let's see how long I can last!" I set a timer for two minutes.

Within seconds of turning the handle, I was immediately overcome with a shock so intense that it literally took my breath away. A thousand needles danced across my skin, and I began hyperventilating. My brain was screaming at me to turn off the water, but I couldn't let myself do it. I wasn't doing *nearly* as well as I thought I would, but my competitive side kicked in.

I can do this. I can go the full two minutes. I'm not going to let this stupid water win. I'm better than this.

For what felt like an eternity, my brain still begging me to hit the eject button, I persevered. When I finally caved and jumped out of the water, I checked my phone to see how long I had lasted.

Twenty seconds.

That's it?! I was flabbergasted. I couldn't imagine how someone could withstand that for a minute, let alone two or three. Yet as awful as that experience was, there was something kind of fun about it. Here I was, in my bathroom, on a random weekday, feeling like I had just overcome an enormous challenge—and my day had barely started.

I vowed to give it another shot the next day, and this time I lasted a bit longer. I kept at it until, within a week or so, three minutes became routine. Immediately I began to notice benefits like improved mental clarity throughout my day and as time went on, an overall improvement in my mood. I felt noticeably more calm and small things that used to annoy me, like getting cut off in traffic, no longer phased me—outside of a racetrack, at least.

If you had told me during that first cold shower that this would be something I would come to look forward to, I would've said you were out of your mind. Yet, I now look forward to this as part of my daily routine—just like I look forward to exercising, eating the right foods, and so on. In my travels, I even get excited at the idea of experiencing *colder* waters than what my home is capable of (Montana and Switzerland currently hold the record).

STRESS: THE GOOD AND THE BAD

In Chapters 3 and 4, we covered the many negative effects that stress can have on your body and brain. As it turns out, some stressors can be beneficial—at least in the right doses. This concept is called **hormesis**, and taking a cold plunge or a cold shower is one example of this in action.

Hormesis (from the Greek word *hormáein*, which means "to excite" or "set in motion") is the biological principle that suggests organisms can adapt to low or moderate doses of environmental or self-imposed stressors, which may be harmful at higher doses. This in turn can improve one's ability to tolerate other challenges, and in some cases improve your overall health and longevity.

Take my cold showers, for example. Short-duration, regular, and intentionally controlled cold exposure can activate beneficial pathways in your body. But prolonged exposure to extreme cold can lead to hypothermia or even death. The key is finding the right balance—enough stress to trigger the adaptive responses, but not so much that it causes harm. This is characterized by what scientists call a "biphasic dose response," where low doses of a given stressor have a beneficial effect while high doses of that same stressor can be harmful or even toxic.

That said, not all stressors are beneficial. As we've covered, chronic stress is decidedly not good for your body or brain. Technostress is also becoming an increasingly common problem, where we experience stress as a result of the endless amount of information being pushed at us through digital means. Unfortunately, most people today experience some level of chronic stress due to circumstances they feel are outside their control, whether it's related to their job, finances, relationships, or any number of other perceived problems. It is a bit ironic to think that our ancestors, who had to worry about getting eaten alive by predators or succumbing to a simple infection, in many ways likely experienced less stress overall than we do today.

In this chapter, we're going to explore the positive and negative attributes of stress. We'll start with the good stressors by explaining why hormetic practices like cold plunges and sauna bathing can be beneficial for your body and brain, as well as how to introduce these interventions safely in your life. Then, we'll talk about how to negate the effects of negative stressors with stress management techniques like digital detoxes and guided breathing.

Hormetic practices and stress management techniques are certainly worth considering for anyone looking to develop a comprehensive longevity framework. Effective stress management is particularly important as it can not only help improve how you feel immediately, but of equal importance, can have a substantial impact on many of the hallmarks of aging we discussed in Chapter 4. And as you'll see, there is some remarkable data around the impact this can have on your current mental and physical performance, as well as your longevity.

Again, every action you take is an investment in your future health, and effectively managing your stress (both the good and the bad) is another important form of this investment.

THE "GOOD" STRESSORS

At the risk of sounding like my drill instructor from officer training, there is some truth to the idea that we've gotten "soft" as humans. (If you were to ask Chief Ruiz, he would say it is unequivocally true based on the performance of his recruits, or lack thereof.)

Throughout human history, your ancestors were regularly exposed to substantial environmental stressors, including situations like extreme temperature changes. There was a time when they simply dealt with those adversities, and their bodies were forced to adapt accordingly. However, since the advent of warm clothing, indoor heating and air conditioning, and climate-controlled automobiles, we spend nearly all our time in what has been termed the **thermoneutral zone**, or the range of ambient temperatures where your body can maintain its core temperature without needing to actively regulate heat production or loss, a process called **thermoregulation**.

By keeping your body in a constant state of comfort, you are actually depriving yourself of the ability to experience some of the positive stressors that activate various longevity pathways in your body. This comfort may feel nice in the short term, but in the long term, it could actually be detrimental to your health and your longevity. Therefore, working small doses of "good" stressors into your daily routine through hormetic practices can be a highly effective tactic at slowing your rate of aging and keeping you more resilient well into your later years.

The most important part of implementing any hormetic practice is towing the line between "healthy" and "dangerous." Sitting in a sauna for twenty minutes, for example, can be a highly effective stressor. Sitting in one for two hours can result in extreme dehydration and can potentially kill you, so this should be approached with caution.

It's also worth noting that not all stressors are beneficial, even in small doses. Ionizing radiation, for example, appears to *only* cause harm without providing any hormetic benefit, regardless of dose. (So don't go stand next to a nuclear reactor and expect to turn into the Incredible Hulk—it will not end well.) The key is identifying the stressors that, when properly dosed, create beneficial adaptations in your body without creating harm.

Some examples of positive stressors include intentional heat exposure, cold exposure, fasting, exercise, red light therapy, and the consumption of phytochemicals. Within each of these categories you may choose to undertake, you'll need to be careful about the timing, duration, and dose of exposure. Given that we've already covered exercise and fasting in previous chapters, I'll skip those here. But just know that those are also technically examples of hormetic stressors, as they both provide a challenging stressor that your body gradually adapts to the more you do them.

For our purposes, we'll be focusing on heat and cold exposure, red light therapy, and phytochemicals, as these have all been proven to provide specific benefits with respect to your immediate and long-term health. That said, there are likely many forms of hormetic stress that can be beneficial. The act of doing "hard things" is typically good for your brain and body, just be sure to stay within safe limits.

One way to think about this is to use the Fun Scale. Rainer Newberry, a geology professor at the University of Alaska Fairbanks, came up with this scale to categorize the types of fun people experience during outdoor adventures, particularly in challenging situations:

- **Type 1 Fun is fun while you're doing it.** The activity is enjoyable and doesn't involve much effort or discomfort. It's fun in the moment and fun when you look back on it.
- **Type 2 Fun is fun in retrospect.** The activity is challenging or uncomfortable, but rewarding and enjoyable afterward. Not always fun in the moment, but fun when you look back on it.
- **Type 3 Fun is not fun at all.** The activity is challenging and uncomfortable, and you would never voluntarily do it again. Not fun in the moment, and not fun when you look back on it.

While slightly comical, this is actually a decent way to categorize hormetic stressors. Type 1 Fun is likely not providing enough of a stressor, Type 2 Fun is likely providing a good amount, and Type 3 Fun is likely too much. For what it's worth, I experienced *plenty* of Type 2 and 3 fun in the military, which make for some good stories.

In addition to the long-term benefits to your health, which may take time to fully appreciate, regular, intentional doses of these controlled types of stress can absolutely provide more resilience in navigating your day. Whether it's an angry email from your boss, an uncomfortable encounter with a stranger, or an argument with your partner, there is a good chance these circumstances will no longer induce the same physical reaction, or at the very least you'll be better equipped to handle them when they arise after exposing yourself to these interventions more frequently.

With that in mind, all hormetic stressors don't have to be miserable, and putting your body through a simulated challenge can provide very tangible rewards afterward!

INTENTIONAL HEAT EXPOSURE (SAUNA)

Of all the hormetic interventions we'll discuss, regular sauna use has perhaps the most robust evidence supporting its benefits for your health and overall longevity. We can thank the Scandinavians for most of this data, as saunas are practically a way of life over there. The Finnish in particular have been using saunas regularly for hundreds of years, and much of the evidence we rely on comes from that part of the world.

Thanks to all that data, regular sauna use has now been linked to a significant reduction in cardiovascular disease, including sudden cardiac death and fatal coronary heart disease. This is thought to take place through multiple mechanisms, including reducing stiffness of the arteries, which helps to lower blood pressure, improves the function of the lining of the blood vessels, decreases inflammation and oxidative stress in the body, and even lowers fats and lipids in the bloodstream—all of which are components of metabolic syndrome, as you may recall.

Regular sauna use also results in the upregulation of what are called *heat shock proteins*. When exposed to heat, your body produces these, which act as "molecular chaperones" that assist in the folding, assembly, and transportation of other normal proteins within your cells. They can also help protect your cells from other external stressors.

One of the hallmarks of aging, as we know, is the loss of proteostasis—the proper balance and function of proteins within your cells. When your proteins become misfolded, they don't function correctly, which can lead to various diseases and accelerated aging as we covered in Chapter 4. Heat shock proteins help maintain proteostasis, essentially keeping your cellular machinery running smoothly and help prevent accelerated aging of your cells.

The research on sauna use is particularly impressive. In studies of Finnish men, those who used a sauna two to three times per week had a 22 percent lower risk of sudden cardiac death compared to those who used it just once weekly. For men who used the sauna four to seven times per week, that risk reduction jumped to an astounding 63 percent.

When it comes to all-cause mortality—dying from any cause—sauna use shows similar benefits. In a study of men who used the sauna two to three times weekly, they experienced a 16 percent lower all-cause mortality, while those using it four to seven times weekly saw a 22 percent reduction. Combining high cardiorespiratory fitness with frequent sauna use resulted in an even more impressive 37 percent reduction in all-cause mortality, which is perhaps no surprise given everything you now know about the benefits of exercise.

Regular sauna use has also been shown to provide stress relief, improve depression scores, lower anxiety, enhance sleep quality, and improve overall mental wellbeing. This is thought to occur through the increase in the same heat shock proteins referenced above, the release of beta-endorphins (which elevate mood), and an increase in BDNF (brain-derived neurotrophic factor), which we know is helpful in slowing the rate of aging of your neurons and improving their overall function.

This all points to sauna use being a valuable tool to combat your risk of neurodegenerative disease, and the numbers appear to back this up. Several studies in fact have demonstrated a whopping 64 percent reduction in the risk of developing dementia for individuals using the sauna four to seven times per week compared to once weekly. Of equal importance, these benefits appear largely equivalent for both men and women, despite the studies referenced above focusing primarily on male participants.

While any statistics should be taken with a grain of salt, in general it appears that regular sauna use is largely beneficial. Research suggests that temperatures between 70–100°C (158–212°F) for a duration of fifteen to twenty minutes confers the greatest benefit. Critically, as many of those statistics alluded to, frequency is key. Four to seven sessions per week seem to provide substantial benefits over infrequent use. It should also be noted that twenty-minute sessions also appear particularly effective relative to shorter durations.

As far as which type of sauna to use, anything that exposes you to the ambient temperatures referenced above should provide a beneficial dose response, with most of the research in this area focusing on traditional Finnish dry saunas. These are what you likely picture when you think of one: a relatively small, confined space with a heater and rocks that can also be doused with a small amount of water to create some steam, but in general have very low humidity. This is because traditional Finnish saunas use dry heat to raise the ambient temperature, which then heats your body indirectly, thereby inducing the changes we've mentioned.

The other two popular ways to receive controlled heat exposure are infrared saunas and steam rooms. As their name implies, infrared saunas use infrared light to heat your body directly, but at much lower ambient temperatures. This type of sauna has become increasingly popular but doesn't yet appear to have the same robust level of evidence as traditional Finnish saunas yet. The same goes for steam rooms, which produce a much higher humidity environment, rather than dry heat. I would argue there is simply not enough evidence at the moment to say for certain that these options are more effective than traditional Finnish saunas, which is what I personally utilize for this reason. The other two likely provide some benefit, it just isn't clear yet to what degree (pun intended).

Like with any hormetic stressor, safety is a must when considering sauna use. It's worth noting that regular sauna use has been shown to reduce sperm count and motility in males, although this appears reversible within six months or less. So, if you and your partner are actively planning for conception, this should be a consideration. Pregnant women and children should also likely avoid sauna use, given differences in their ability to effectively regulate body temperature, which may be impacted by prolonged ambient heat exposure. As with any new health practice, always consult with your personal healthcare provider before beginning, especially if you have any underlying health conditions.

INTENTIONAL COLD EXPOSURE

If you went back to 1995 and told someone that you liked to dunk yourself into ice cold water every morning for health benefits, they would've looked at you like you were from another planet. Nowadays, it's a fairly normal practice. Intentional cold exposure has recently surged in popularity, with "cold plunges" and ice baths becoming increasingly common. And while the evidence for longevity from cold exposure isn't as robust as for sauna use, there are still several documented benefits worth considering.

To be clear, cold exposure *has* been demonstrated to increase lifespan in invertebrates like worms (C. elegans), fruit flies (Drosophila), and microscopic organisms called rotifers. However, the effect in higher-order mammals, including humans, appears less pronounced and more variable. Given the current evidence available, we can't definitively say that cold exposure extends human lifespan yet.

That said, cold exposure does offer several substantial health benefits, in particular with respect to metabolic health. Studies have shown that exposure to ambient air temperatures between 16–19°C (61–66°F) for one to two hours daily over ten days to six weeks can increase the quantity of what is called brown adipose tissue (BAT) by up to 45 percent and its oxidative metabolism by more than twofold.

Brown adipose tissue differs from regular white fat in that it's rich in mitochondria (giving it a brown appearance under a microscope, hence the name) and is therefore highly metabolically active. Unlike white fat, which primarily stores energy, brown fat burns energy to produce heat. This increase in BAT can raise your basal metabolic rate—how many calories you burn at rest—which has been shown to help with weight management and improve insulin sensitivity and glucose metabolism, particularly in people with obesity or type 2 diabetes. Therefore, this *may* improve human longevity by helping to avoid metabolic dysfunction, but no clear data exists yet to prove this for certain.

Now, this type of cold exposure is very different from intentional water exposure in terms of intensity and duration. The former is more like spending time outdoors without a jacket when it's a little chilly for an hour or two a day, assuming you can mimic this type of environment. This is probably more practical in the fall or spring when temperatures are consistently in this range but is of course dependent upon where you live and your local climate. What I take away from this is that it's probably worth being slightly less comfortable in this type of environment while you're spending time outdoors, but don't overdo it.

Taking a cold plunge or cold shower does still confer its own benefits. However. cold showers at about 20°C (68°F) for two to three minutes have been shown to improve mood, reduce symptoms of depression and anxiety, and decrease mental fatigue. This is believed to result from activation of the sympathetic nervous system (your "fight or flight" mode) which increases levels of beta-endorphins and norepinephrine—neurotransmitters that can improve your mood and mental clarity.

Furthermore, there is some evidence that cold exposure lowers inflammation and helps combat oxidative stress within the body, which might have some anti-aging effects when we consider the hallmarks of aging. Between this, an increased metabolism, and increased mitochondrial biogenesis, there may well be a significantly positive impact on the hallmarks of aging, although yet there doesn't appear to be a proven reduction in all-cause mortality or lifespan extension.

It is worth noting that cold exposure does increase your core body temperature, as we discussed in Chapter 7 and the impact this can have on your sleep. When exposed to cold, your blood vessels in the periphery constrict, shunting blood to your core to protect your vital organs. This raises your core temperature and increases alertness, which can be beneficial in the morning but potentially counterproductive before bedtime when your body naturally needs to lower its core temperature to prepare for quality sleep.

Another consideration for anyone looking to gain muscle size is that cold water immersion post-exercise has been shown to blunt mTOR signaling, which decreases muscle hypertrophy (growth). While this doesn't appear to substantially impact strength gains, those specifically looking to increase muscle mass might want to time their cold exposure away from their workouts, perhaps beforehand for an additional energy boost.

Cold exposure has also been shown to increase the activity of SIRT6, a protein in the sirtuin family known to improve DNA repair. SIRT6 is involved in chromatin maintenance, tumor suppression, and anti-aging mechanisms via glucose regulation and NAD+ balance, which may be further preliminary evidence still for its potential longevity benefits.

And last but certainly not least, safety is paramount with cold exposure. Overexposure can induce hypothermia, which can be dangerous or even fatal. Cold exposure can also temporarily impair immune system function, which could increase infection risk, especially in elderly populations. Your body is generally pretty good at telling you when you need to get out of the cold; however, you need to be very mindful of this regardless for your own safety. I can say from experience that it certainly will tell you to get out of the cold when you first start performing cold plunges. The first time can be quite a shock, but it does get easier over time and can even become an enjoyable part of your day with noticeable benefits!

PHYTOCHEMICALS

Phytochemicals are naturally occurring bioactive compounds found in plants that can initiate mild, beneficial cellular stress responses that enhance your cells' resistance to other more severe stressors. While they could be considered part of our nutrition discussion, they also function as hormetic stressors, which makes them relevant to this chapter. These compounds—which include flavonoids, carotenoids, and phenolic compounds—exhibit antioxidant properties that can help reduce oxidative stress and inflammation in the body. This can potentially mitigate chronic diseases such as cardiovascular disease, cancer, diabetes, and neurodegenerative conditions like Alzheimer's.

Phytochemicals modulate specific cellular processes including cell proliferation (or division and growth), apoptosis (programmed cell death), and regulation of microRNAs, which are important for proper gene expression. They also promote healthy gut bacteria while inhibiting harmful strains, which can enhance nutrient absorption and further lower inflammation throughout your body.

One key mechanism is their ability to act as "chemical chaperones" that also promote proper protein folding and prevent misfolding or aggregation of abnormal proteins, which you may recognize also results in a loss of proteostasis. While heat shock proteins from sauna bathing help maintain proteostasis through a temperature-dependent pathway, phytochemicals achieve similar results through a chemical pathway.

When you consume these compounds in plants, they trigger adaptive responses within your cells, which leads to the production of protective proteins and antioxidant enzymes that keep your cells healthy. This mild chemical stress therefore ultimately makes your cells more resilient to other external stressors and may slow various aspects of cellular aging.

You can find phytochemicals in a variety of brightly colored fruits and vegetables, including:

- Spinach, kale, and collard greens
- Carrots, beets, and pumpkins
- Tomatoes and red onions
- Berries (especially blueberries and strawberries)
- Whole grains
- Cruciferous vegetables (broccoli, cauliflower)
- Beans, nuts, and seeds
- Tea (especially green tea)
- Dark chocolate

The simplest way to incorporate phytochemicals into your diet is to "eat the rainbow." There isn't an exact recommended dosage, but eating a wide variety of fruits, vegetables, legumes, and whole grains will likely be enough to achieve the benefits of this particular family of hormetic stressors.

RED LIGHT THERAPY

Red light therapy involves exposing the skin or other tissues to red or near-infrared light. Originally investigated by NASA to improve wound healing for astronauts in space, with the right application this therapy has shown benefits for skin health, eye conditions, and potentially other processes. Too much red light could theoretically be harmful, which is why this also falls into the hormesis category—getting the "right amount" is important.

Red light therapy works through a process called *photobiomodulation,* where exposure near-infrared light (typically 630–1,000nm wavelength) stimulates certain cellular processes. For example, when this light penetrates your skin or retinal cells, it can enhance mitochondrial function by upregulating genes involved in mitochondrial energy production (in particular by acting on a protein complex called cytochrome c oxidase, which helps produce more ATP).

Red light therapy is most commonly used on skin, either for improving overall skin health, treating specific skin conditions like acne, or healing wounds. For this application in particular, red light therapy has been shown to:

- Reverse UV-induced damage by enhancing DNA repair through a process called base excision repair
- Reduce oxidative stress and increase ATP production within the mitochondria of skin cells, thereby keeping them younger
- Increase collagen and elastin production, maintaining skin elasticity, and reducing the appearance of wrinkles

- Stimulate fibroblasts, which produce collagen in the skin, which helps keep a more youthful appearance

Many users report noticeable improvements to their skin within days to weeks of consistent use. I can say anecdotally that I've used red light therapy to help heal wounds and been impressed with the results—the healing process does appear noticeably faster, but there are certainly a number of potential biases at play here.

Eye health is another area where red light therapy shows promise. It has demonstrated improvements in age-related macular degeneration by enhancing retinal cell mitochondrial function. There's also emerging evidence that it may help with myopia (nearsightedness). And yes, this does mean shining a red light into your eyes—it might go against everything you thought you knew about eye health, but it does not cause damage in the same way UV light or blue light from a screen could (which has actually been shown to *decrease* mitochondrial function).

The research on red light therapy for brain health is somewhat more contentious due to the challenge of light penetration. Red light can only penetrate tissue to a depth of several millimeters, which means it easily reaches the skin and retina but has difficulty reaching deeper structures like the brain. However, in animal models, red light therapy has shown promise for reducing neuroinflammation and improving recovery from traumatic brain injury. As of this writing, human clinical trials for using red light therapy to treat Alzheimer's disease are currently underway, although more research for its definitive impact on this condition are needed.

There are some claims of red light therapy healing joint pain and injuries, but I would also approach this with a degree of cautious skepticism for similar reasons. It is unlikely that LED-based red light is able to penetrate deep enough to affect joints unless a more concentrated, higher-energy beam could do so, which is currently another topic of investigation. Quality human data as of this writing are lacking, which may change.

There is, however, emerging data on the impact of red light therapy on metabolic health. Recent studies have shown that exposure after meals has reduced peak blood glucose elevation, which may again be due to increased mitochondrial activity, which is where the majority of glucose metabolism takes place. While more studies are also needed here, this may provide yet another layer of benefit for longevity through maintaining steady glucose levels.

The optimal dose for red light therapy isn't entirely clear from current research, but ten to thirty minutes of exposure two to five times per week appears to be both safe and effective at least for skin and eye applications. This is typically done through red-light blankets or mats (for the body), red-light masks (for the face), or red-light glasses (for the eyes).

Red light therapy is generally considered very safe, as this part of the light spectrum doesn't cause DNA damage like ultraviolet, X-ray, or gamma radiation (unless your name is Bruce Banner). It's important to note that while red light therapy is beneficial, blue light (which is prevalent in screens and many indoor LED lights) may have opposite effects, potentially inactivating cytochrome C oxidase and potentially accelerating aging. Yikes.

If you've been wondering about the efficacy of interventions like cold plunges or saunas, I hope that by now you can see there is real evidence showing how these methods can positively impact your health and longevity. By introducing the right challenges in controlled, intentional ways, you can kickstart many of the adaptive pathways in your body that your ancestors once relied upon, but which are now less readily available given the comforts of modern life. When used appropriately, these, as the data suggests, have the potential to slow the aging process and offer a host of other short- and long-term benefits.

In addition to the four methods we've just discussed, this general concept also applies to other areas like exercise and intermittent fasting. Exposing your body to the right kind of stress is typically beneficial in the right doses. It's also worth noting that your body is pretty good at telling you when you're doing too much. If you experience significant pain while exercising, for example, that's probably a sign you should stop and make sure you haven't suffered an injury. If you choose to undertake any of these methods, listen to your body. A little bit of discomfort is good, and a sign that you are very likely triggering the right responses, but a lot of discomfort could be a sign that something is wrong.

As we move into the negative stressors, this distinction becomes a bit less black and white, as most of the negative stressors we experience in our daily lives result in low levels of chronic stress. Although this type of stress *can* cause physical symptoms, it often goes unnoticed or is simply thought to be just a fact of life. Whether you realize it or not, the daily stressors you experience from work, technology, or just "life" in general *are* likely having an impact on your health and longevity—but they can be effectively managed.

THE "BAD STRESSORS" (AND HOW TO MANAGE THEM)

While hormetic stressors can substantially benefit your health when properly applied, chronic "negative" stress presents a significant threat to both your immediate wellbeing and long-term health. This concept is very similar to what we've previously discussed about inflammation—helpful in small doses, but harmful when incurred over a long period of time, even at low levels.

When you experience chronic stress, your sympathetic nervous system—the "fight or flight" response—remains constantly engaged, which can cause problems. While this helped your ancestors evade predators and safely react to dangerous situations, it's no longer of much use when you encounter minor stressors like an annoying email or a particularly frustrating commute, which are ever present throughout your day. Even these seemingly minor events can have significant repercussions on your brain and body over the long term.

Unfortunately, this has become an inevitable part of life for the vast majority of our society. Rather than spending your effort trying to eliminate this constant barrage of stress, however, which would be virtually impossible, I would encourage you to start by accepting reality for what it is. Know that stressful events are going to happen, but rather than letting them control you, you can learn how to control your *interpretation* of them, and therefore, your response. In Chapter 2, we learned that your brain can attach meaning to any given situation, which means that through the process of neuroplasticity you can absolutely control your response to stressful situations. Learning how to do that is perhaps the most effective way to minimize or negate the effects of stress in your life.

HOW CHRONIC STRESS AFFECTS YOUR BODY AND BRAIN

When you experience acute stress, there are a number of rapid physiologic changes that take place in your body. At a high level, when your brain perceives an external as a threat to your safety, your hypothalamus then cues your adrenal glands to immediately release epinephrine and norepinephrine into your bloodstream. Your body then transforms into fight-or flight-mode, which triggers an instant cascade of effects—your heart rate and blood pressure elevate, your pupils dilate, your muscles tense, your rate of breathing increases, and you may even start to sweat depending on the severity of the situation.

These are all largely beneficial if you are in fact facing a real threat to your safety, like having to avoid an oncoming car or being chased by a large animal. But given what we already know about the primary threats and hallmarks of aging, we are not designed to keep this system turned on over the long term. Over time, chronic stress can lead to serious health problems like increased risk of cardiovascular disease and neurodegenerative disease, a weakened immune system, disrupted sleep problems, impaired digestion, and increased inflammation. Generally speaking, chronic stress accelerates cellular aging throughout your body.

On a more immediate front, stress can also impact your cognitive function. When your body is in a stressed state, you cannot effectively use your prefrontal cortex—the part of your brain responsible for higher-level thinking, planning, and purposeful action. Instead, you operate from your more primitive limbic system, which prioritizes survival over long-term thinking. This is often why people freeze up on stage and can't remember what they've spent days preparing to discuss. This system is quite powerful.

This also means when you remain chronically stressed, you are more likely to default to what's easiest and most comforting in the moment whether you realize it or not. Your brain is very adept at making you feel comfortable and secure, even when the outside world does not appear that way. Therefore, it can naturally guide you to mechanisms to help you escape the painful reality of stress, whether those result in healthy behaviors or not. Very often this can look like turning to sugar-sweetened beverages, savory fast foods, and scrolling mindlessly through social media or your TV series of choice in an effort to make you feel better. This is one major way chronic stress can lead to consistently poor nutrition choices, missed workouts, and even disrupted sleep—essentially undermining your adherence to all the critical interventions we've discussed so far.

This is problematic on its own, but what makes it even more challenging is how quickly this can create a snowball effect, as neuroplasticity works both ways and dopamine is a powerful catalyst in shaping behavior. For example, if you're constantly stressed at work, the quality of your work will likely suffer, which likely translates to even more stress when your boss becomes upset with you. This might even cause some sleepless nights in anticipation of the additional pressure you face, which only incurs more stress, and you wake up unrested the next day, further hindering your work performance. With so much going on, it's even harder to set aside time to exercise and you're more likely to default to a quick meal for comfort over a nutritious one. All of this can then lead to even more stress, which only exacerbates the problems you were experiencing in the first place, and round and round it goes. Sound familiar?

While you're in the middle of that whole mess, there's also an endless flow of information being pushed at you through all the various screens and devices in your life. This constant stimulus alone creates its own persistent source of stress that your body also wasn't designed to handle—which only adds another layer. I'm honestly getting stressed just writing about this!

The good news is, there are plenty of evidence-based techniques to effectively combat this—but before we get into those, I have a quick and slightly embarrassing confession to make. While writing this book, I had initially forgotten to include stress management techniques in Part 2 (originally, this chapter only included hormesis). During the book edits, I realized my mistake and adjusted this chapter to include both hormesis *and* stress management.

However, for the sake of brevity (and to lower my own stress levels and those of my editors), I've chosen to include most of the "how-to" content for stress mitigation techniques online. So, as you read through the interventions below, I would absolutely encourage you to head to the resource page at TranscendHealthGroup.com/Resources to download the accompanying free PDF, which provides more instructional guidance on each of them.

As a bonus, having this in digital form allows me to update the information more regularly—so depending on when you're reading this, you may find even more up-to-date content online. While it didn't make the final cut for the book, I told my editors I would absolutely not compromise on providing maximum value to my readers (you), so please take me up on that offer and I hope it offers even more perspective.

The longer I'm around, the more experiences I have that remind me of my humanness and the fact that we all make mistakes, and I believe we should be more gracious with ourselves in moments like these. I view life as a series of moments that create either wins or opportunities to improve. While publishing my first book is definitely in the win column, the overlooked omission serves as the latter and is one more opportunity to improve upon when it comes time to write my second.

EVIDENCE-BASED STRESS MANAGEMENT TECHNIQUES

Chances are, you're aware of some of the most common ways to manage stress. Techniques like yoga, breathwork, and meditation are all commonly known to alleviate stress, for example. While these are absolutely beneficial, I would also keep in mind that stress management doesn't necessarily have to be a rigid part of your routine, like exercise.

Many of these techniques can be easily implemented as needed throughout your day, like doing a quick stretch at your desk or thinking of something you're grateful for. Hopefully, by reading this chapter and experimenting with some of these interventions, you'll also start to become more aware of moments in your life when you're feeling stressed. Even just taking a few deep breaths at times like this can help you regain your composure, improving your immediate performance and long-term health in the process.

Here are some of the most effective methods, according to current data. Remember that you can find more details on how to implement these on the resource page.

BREATHWORK

Breathwork is perhaps the most immediate and accessible stress management tool for everyone. Various breathing techniques have been shown to directly engage the parasympathetic nervous system, which is essentially the opposite of the fight-or flight-response.

The physiological sigh is one such particularly effective technique. This involves a deep, slow, full inhalation through your nose to completely fill your lungs. Once you feel like you can't get any more air in, you then take a second, brief, sharp inhale, also through the nose, and then slowly let it all go through the mouth. This type of breath triggers a reflex that engages your parasympathetic nervous system, instantly helping you shift from stressed to calm. What makes breathwork especially valuable is that it's available anywhere, at any time, and requires no special equipment.

Box breathing is also a simple technique you can employ to lower stress. It involves a slow inhalation through your nose over four seconds, holding your breath in for four seconds, exhaling through your mouth over four seconds, then holding your exhale for four seconds. If you can imagine four equal sides to your breathing, it would look like a square or box. This is a common technique taught to special forces soldiers to maintain their parasympathetic tone in the middle of combat and therefore keep their judgment and levelheadedness in top shape.

MINDFULNESS MEDITATION

Mindfulness meditation is another proven stress-reduction technique with substantial evidence supporting its benefits. This involves focusing your awareness on the present, paying attention to your thoughts, feelings, and sensations. From personal experience, I can say this is initially more challenging than you might think—but the more you do it, the better you'll get.

Regular practice has been shown to reduce cortisol levels, decrease inflammation, and improve emotional regulation. Even brief periods of mindfulness meditation—just a few minutes daily—can help calm your nervous system and reset your stress response. For those with more time, twenty to thirty-minute sessions provide even greater benefits. There are many ways to do this, including guided meditations, group sessions, and apps.

PRACTICING GRATITUDE

In Chapter 2, we learned how positive psychology can actually transform your brain. One way of implementing this in your life is to practice gratitude on a regular basis. Simply taking a moment out of your day to think about all the things you're grateful for can make a noticeable difference in your outlook and lower stress levels throughout your day.

Another way to incorporate this into your life is to change your perspective from "I have to" to "I get to." This has been incredibly powerful in my own life. Take this book, for example. There are times where I dread opening my laptop to work on this, knowing the amount of focus and effort it will take. But then I'll stop myself.

No one is forcing me to write this book. This is not something I *have* to do. Really, the fact that I'm in a position where I can spend my time on such a creative endeavor is an incredible gift. I *get* to write this book! I am blessed to have that opportunity. How awesome is that? Simply shifting my mindset in this way has helped me through many aspects of life, and I've heard the same from many of our Transcend Health community members.

This simple mindset shift activates different neural pathways and can significantly reduce your perception of stress. Beyond the immediate psychological benefits, gratitude practices have been linked to longer lifespans, improved sleep quality, and enhanced immune function. People who regularly practice gratitude even live longer, which is pretty amazing!

EARLY MORNING LIGHT EXPOSURE

We already know that morning sunlight exposure helps set your circadian rhythm, which regulates your sleep-wake cycle, but as you may recall it can also be helpful in managing stress. Getting ten to fifteen minutes of early morning sunlight has been shown to improve resilience to stress. The additional benefits of improved mood, enhanced mental clarity, and sleep also likely reduce stress, creating a positive feedback loop.

STRATEGIC EXERCISE

While we've already covered exercise extensively in Chapter 5, it's worth highlighting its role as a stress management tool. Morning exercise in particular can be helpful in managing stress throughout the day.

Exercise stimulates blood flow to the brain, enhances memory formation, elevates BDNF levels, activates various pathways in the brain and body that enhance longevity, and helps maintain healthy blood glucose levels—all of which keep you sharp and better able to combat stress throughout the day. Studies also consistently demonstrate that regular exercise leads to improvements in symptoms of depression and anxiety while enhancing overall mood, which can also impact stress levels.

TIME MANAGEMENT

How you structure your day can significantly impact your stress levels. Research suggests that working in ninety-minute intervals with intentional breaks of ten to fifteen minutes provides optimal cognitive function while minimizing stress. This pattern of focused work followed by intentional breaks mirrors the natural ultradian rhythms of your brain, which cycle between higher and lower energy roughly every ninety minutes.

During these breaks, it's important to shift gears and do something else. Going outside, moving your body, and changing your environment are particularly powerful—but whatever you can do to "reset" mentally should provide a benefit.

This is another situation where you may experience a positive feedback loop. If you're really busy, you might think it's better to keep working than take a fifteen-minute break, but sticking with these ninety-minute intervals will likely boost your productivity overall, which should ultimately lower your stress as you'll have less to do and less on your mind to worry about.

DIGITAL DETOX

Deliberately limiting screen time and digital work can significantly lower anxiety and allow your brain to calm down from the constant influx of information. This is especially important in the evenings when screen exposure can interfere with your sleep. By creating boundaries around technology use, you create space for your nervous system to calm down and return to a state of balance.

There are many ways to conduct a "digital detox" but it's worth noting that even short periods away from screens can provide meaningful relief from technostress. While you may think of a digital detox as some big event where you cut screens out of your life for days or weeks at a time, it doesn't have to be that extreme. Simply taking breaks or minimizing screen time in general can be helpful.

ANALYZING YOUR SCHEDULE

One powerful but often overlooked technique is to systematically analyze your current schedule. I like to do this by opening a note on my phone writing down my daily schedule, getting as granular as possible from the moment I wake up to the moment I go to bed. I'll then take a step back and study my day.

When I do this, I often find inefficiencies and stressful points in my routine. I can then reorganize my schedule to alleviate those problems. I can also use this as a chance to incorporate regular breaks and movement throughout my day, ensuring I actually do them instead of getting sucked into my work. Equally importantly is to leave protected time off—time to think, reflect, exercise, spend time with your family, or do anything you enjoy. As strange as it sounds to schedule time for fun, this should really be the first thing you do, and everything else should come second.

I know this sounds overly simple, but if you've never tried it, you might be surprised by what you find. Considering giving it a shot and revisiting your schedule every now and then. This is a great way to not only lower stress but just make your day-to-day life a little easier and more enjoyable. There are even a handful of tools that now help with this, in particular those that make great use of AI, which make this process even more stress-free and far simpler.

THE BALANCING ACT

Throughout this chapter, we've explored both sides of the stress equation—the beneficial hormetic stressors that can strengthen you when properly applied and the harmful chronic stressors that accelerate aging and disease when left unchecked. Interestingly, this brings up an important point to keep in mind throughout your longevity journey: the idea of balance.

Excess stress can absolutely cause problems, but no stress at all isn't great either. The same could be said for many of the previously mentioned interventions. Overactivation of mTOR can be problematic, but so can too much AMPK. Morning sun exposure can be helpful, but prolonged exposure to UV rays can cause cellular senescence, telomere dysfunction, and increased risk of cancer.

The phrase "everything in moderation" does hold some merit as we think about our health and longevity. If you choose to implement any of the interventions in this book, I encourage you again to prioritize consistency over intensity. Start small, build gradually, and listen to your body's signals. What works for someone else may not work for you, and that's perfectly normal. The goal is to find your personal balance between beneficial challenge and necessary recovery.

If you haven't already, be sure to head to the resource page at TranscendHealthGroup.com/Resources for more information on the stress management techniques we just covered. You'll also find another cheat sheet for this chapter, covering all the specific targets for each intervention so you can keep things in balance.

As we turn our attention to supplements in the next chapter, we'll explore how some vital micronutrients can have a significant impact on your health and longevity over time. Like with so many of our interventions, many of these supplements can also impact your stress levels and in some cases even alleviate the negative effects stress has on your body. It's all interrelated. Remember: each step is an investment in your future self.

KEY TAKEAWAYS

1. **Beneficial stress strengthens while chronic stress weakens.** Hormetic stressors like sauna use, cold exposure, and phytochemicals activate longevity pathways when properly dosed, while unmanaged chronic stress accelerates aging and undermines health. Understanding this distinction is key for optimizing your stress response.

2. **Consistency trumps intensity in both hormetic practices and stress management.** Regular exposure to moderate hormetic challenges provides greater benefits than occasional intense sessions, and the same principle applies to stress management techniques. Small, sustainable daily practices yield the most powerful long-term results.

3. **Balancing challenge and recovery optimize resilience.** The most effective longevity approach combines both controlled hormetic stressors and intentional stress reduction techniques. This balanced approach helps strengthen your body's adaptive systems while preventing the damage caused by persistent negative stress.

You can find lists of all the specific interventions from this chapter in the Hormesis & Stress Management Cheat Sheets at TranscendHealth Group.com/Resources.

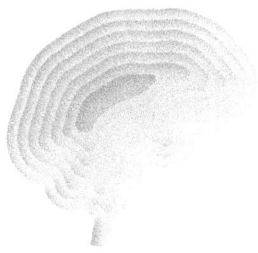

CHAPTER 9
SUPPLEMENTS

AS I ENTERED the exam room, I said hello to Peter and his wife. Having read his chart beforehand, I already knew Peter was here because of concerns about his recent memory loss. On paper, it looked like he may have been experiencing the early stages of dementia. To be sure, I needed more information.

"So, what's been happening with Peter?" I asked. His wife answered.

"Well, I've just been noticing that Peter seems to be a bit more forgetful recently. He now gets lost driving around the neighborhood where we've lived for thirty years, and sometimes he asks the same question multiple times, even when I've just given him the answer. It's strange, and I'm really worried about him. This isn't the Peter I know." Peter looked on glumly.

"I'm so sorry to hear that. How long has this been happening?"

"I don't know, maybe over the last week or so," his wife replied.

"Okay." I sensed she may not have been telling the whole truth. "So just to be clear, there was no strange behavior before that?"

"Well...now that you mention it, I suppose his memory has been slipping for a few months...."

As I continued to ask similar questions from different angles, the timeline seemed to shift. It soon became clear that these problems had been developing for the better part of a year. This gradual onset is typical for many neurodegenerative diseases, which pointed again to my initial concern for dementia.

Peter had never had any imaging or comprehensive lab work done, so the first course of action was to do a thorough workup including a brain MRI and metabolic panel. His MRI came back normal, and most of his metabolic panel looked fine except for one glaring abnormality. Despite the lab registering this as being within the normal range, his vitamin B12 level was alarmingly low at around 230 picograms per milliliter. Peter wasn't just a little deficient—his levels were low enough to cause neurological symptoms, including memory loss that can mimic dementia.

When I asked about his diet, the picture became clearer. Peter primarily ate processed foods and frozen dinners with very little fresh meat, eggs, fish, or animal products of any kind—all excellent sources of B12. There was a chance he was experiencing a neurodegenerative process, which would be extremely difficult to treat, but there was also a chance that his B12 levels could be seriously impairing his memory. Therefore, his B12 levels had to be corrected before I could consider an alternate diagnosis.

We immediately started Peter on B12 injections and worked with his wife to improve his diet. Within months, his cognitive function had returned to normal and the memory problems he was experiencing had practically vanished. His wife told me it was like she had her husband back, and they were thrilled to know that he did not, in fact, have Alzheimer's, which was a major fear of theirs having lost several friends to the disease.

Peter's story is an extreme example of the power of supplements, and what can happen when your body experiences certain micronutrient deficiencies for long periods of time. Peter had likely been deficient in vitamin B12 for years prior to our meeting, but his body was able to store it for several years, until he eventually ran out. When that happens, you can no longer operate critical systems such as making new red blood cells or keeping your neurons healthy. Once that tipping point occurs, problems appear.

In most cases, supplements will not change your life overnight like they did with Peter's, but they can absolutely change the course of your life over time. Your body is remarkably adaptable and can compensate for nutritional deficiencies for years or even decades before the first problem ever becomes apparent. By the time symptoms emerge, the underlying damage may be substantial and is often irreversible. In Peter's case, he was lucky. Others are not.

If you've spent any amount of time in the health and wellness space, especially online, you've likely encountered an endless list of supplements you "should" be taking. Many of these seem to come in and out of fashion and promise remarkable, even life-changing results.

But are these supplements really worth taking? Are there any adverse effects? And of all the supplements out there, which ones do you actually *need* to be taking? These are all valid questions, and the answers can be difficult to find. While some supplements are backed by solid scientific evidence, others make claims that far exceed what current research supports. Unfortunately, there are many companies out there pushing products promising any number of benefits without any validated science behind them. Not to mention, supplements are not regulated by the FDA, so you need to exercise extreme caution when investigating what you are putting in your body.

The placebo effect is also powerful. If you spend a lot of money on a supplement with the expectation that it will change some part of your life because that's what it says on the bottle, chances are you might feel better in some way. But that doesn't necessarily mean *the product* is helping your body on a cellular level.

In this chapter we're going to answer some of the common questions around supplements by looking at what the evidence says. Rather than providing an exhaustive list of every supplement known to man, I've chosen to focus on a handful of supplements that likely apply to the average person and have legitimate evidence that support considering their use for enhancing your longevity. At this point, it should probably go without saying that by no means is this list compulsory. I am merely looking to provide you with a basic understanding of what some of these supplements are, how they work in your body, and how they might fit into an overall longevity framework.

I'd also like to set some expectations. Supplements are, by definition, *supplementary*. Outside of extreme examples like Peter's B12 deficiency, most supplements will likely not change your life overnight and they are by no means a replacement for an intentionally designed healthy lifestyle. Supplements are an excellent way to enhance the foundational pillars of exercise, nutrition, sleep, and stress management. While I am personally optimistic about the direction research in this field is headed, until we have a steady source of reliable, quality evidence, I am not one to get overly excited about supplements *on their own*. I *am* one to get overly excited about exercise and sleep, as you've seen. And let's be real, who doesn't love their sleep?

With that out of the way, let's first talk about what a supplement actually is.

WHAT IS A SUPPLEMENT?

A supplement is something taken by mouth or added to your diet to support your health—typically because you can't or don't receive enough of it from your regular diet. Most supplements are designed to supply your body with additional micronutrients. In Chapter 5 we discussed the three main macronutrients: protein, fat, and carbohydrates (fiber). Those make up the bulk of our nutrition (hence "macro"), whereas micronutrients make up the vitamins and minerals that your body requires (typically in very small amounts) to maintain optimal function. As your body does not produce the majority of these, they must be obtained from your diet in some form.

Ideally, you would receive all the macro and micronutrients you need from a mostly plant-based, whole food, non-processed, and balanced diet (to any of the carnivores reading this, take a deep breath... it's going to be okay). In reality, this is simply not the case for most people. It's extremely difficult, if not impossible, to achieve optimal nutrition given the modifications to our food supply and the availability of quality food in our everyday lives.

According to current estimates, approximately half of the US population and more than two billion people worldwide are deficient in at least one micronutrient. This is a staggering number that highlights just how common nutritional gaps are, even in developed countries with abundant food supplies.

SUPPLEMENTS TO CONSIDER

In the following pages, I will cover some of what I believe to be the highest-yield, evidence-backed supplements, which are generally recognized as safe at the recommended dosages. If you're interested in a more personalized approach or have concerns about the levels of specific micronutrients in your body, testing can be helpful but it may not paint the full picture. Only a few of these micronutrients can currently be accurately assessed via bloodwork—notably, vitamins D and B12—and others, like magnesium for example, may not provide precise or worthwhile data.

I should also again point out (for my US audience) that supplements are not regulated by the FDA in the same way that prescription medications are. This means the quality, purity, and even the actual contents inside the pills you buy can vary dramatically from one brand to another. Rather than suggesting specific brand names, I would simply recommend investigating any company's track record before purchasing from them. Most reputable companies also allow their products to undergo rigorous independent third-party testing to ensure purity and quality. This information should be readily available on their website or upon request.

As you read, keep in mind that you can download the full supplement cheat sheet at TranscendHealthGroup.com/Resources, which we do our best to keep up to date dosage targets for each of the supplements listed.

Look for the labels **GMP** (Good Manufacturing Practices) or **USP** (USP Dietary Supplement Verification program) when considering which supplements to take. These are usually a good indicator of quality, but regardless, be sure to do your due diligence.

MAGNESIUM

Magnesium is an abundant mineral in the body, with the majority stored within your bones. It's estimated that between 50–75 percent of Americans are deficient in magnesium—a surprisingly high number for such a crucial nutrient. What makes magnesium particularly tricky is that accurate levels are actually very difficult to measure.

Because the majority of magnesium in your body is stored in your bones, the amount of magnesium in your blood doesn't always tell the full story. A blood test can measure the amount of magnesium *currently circulating in your bloodstream,* but it doesn't provide an accurate picture of how much magnesium is in your body as a whole. Therefore, you may appear to have sufficient levels in your blood but an insufficient reservoir in the rest of your body. In that case, you would likely be overall deficient in magnesium even though your blood levels appear normal, and odds are you may well be. Over time, magnesium deficiency can lead to serious problems with bone health and many other systems throughout your body.

Magnesium is a cofactor in *more than 300 enzymatic reactions* in your body and is required by every one of your organ systems. Among its many functions, magnesium helps regulate:

- Protein synthesis
- Muscle and nerve function
- Heart rhythm
- Blood glucose control
- Blood pressure
- And many other essential processes

At a cellular level, magnesium is required for energy production, including oxidative phosphorylation and glycolysis—the two main mechanisms by which you make ATP, the primary energy currency in your cells. It's also required for the synthesis of DNA, RNA, and the antioxidant glutathione, which is essential for combating cellular aging by neutralizing harmful free radicals.

While the evidence is mixed, adequate magnesium supplementation has been associated with a 3–10 percent reduction in all-cause mortality. At very high doses, side effects can include gastrointestinal symptoms, weakness, and heart rhythm issues. However, considering most people are likely deficient, these side effects are rarely encountered at recommended doses.

The typically recommended supplementation varies depending on overall levels in your body, but a good starting point tends to be around 300mg per day for women and 400mg per day for men, which is largely based on body mass index. The forms magnesium glycinate and gluconate confer similar benefits, have high bioavailability in the body, and are available over the counter. Magnesium threonate more readily crosses the blood brain barrier and therefore may be a good choice for cognitive health, and magnesium citrate in particular can be used as a laxative so keep that in mind if it's not an intended effect.

Bioavailability refers to the proportion of a drug or other substance which enters the circulation when introduced into the body and is therefore able to have an active effect.

VITAMIN D

Vitamin D is a fat-soluble vitamin that helps with many different mechanisms inside your body and is primarily naturally obtained through sun exposure. It's mostly known for helping maintain calcium and phosphorus levels in the blood, which are necessary for healthy bones and teeth. However, beyond bone health, vitamin D provides numerous other benefits:

- Supports normal immune system function and helps defend against harmful pathogens
- Reduces inflammation throughout the body
- Modulates cell growth, neuromuscular function, and glucose metabolism

- Regulates proteins governing cell proliferation, differentiation, and apoptosis
- Helps regulate blood pressure
- Strengthens muscle fibers and provides cardioprotective effects
- May improve mood, concentration, and memory
- Potentially reduces cognitive decline when maintained at optimal levels

An estimated 35–42 percent of the US population is deficient in vitamin D, although this number is much higher in individuals with darker skin pigmentation—nearly double, in fact. This is largely because melanin in the skin naturally absorbs some of the UV rays needed for vitamin D production.

A deficiency in vitamin D can lead to osteomalacia (softening of the bones) and osteoporosis (low bone mineral density). Both conditions can predispose you to fractures in the event of a fall or trauma. If you remember from our previous chapters, hip fractures in older adults can have mortality rates as high as 58 percent within the first year. Vitamin D is a great tool to help prevent those fractures from happening in the first place. Some studies have also demonstrated a 7–20 percent reduction in all-cause mortality for individuals with optimal levels of vitamin D, which is perhaps no surprise given its array of functions.

As you're probably aware, you can achieve adequate vitamin D production from the sun. Even just ten minutes of midday sun exposure to uncovered skin can help your body produce the required levels. The relationship between vitamin D levels and skin cancer remains somewhat unclear, however, so it would be advisable to use a mineral-based sunscreen for protection if spending extended time outdoors, especially for fair-skinned individuals. That said, if you live in a climate with frequent overcast or shorter days, supplementation might be a good idea. The best way to know where you stand, of course, is by getting tested.

The general recommended supplementation is usually between 1,500–2,000 IU per day, though this varies depending on total levels in the body, which can be accurately assessed via bloodwork. Because vitamin D is fat-soluble, its stores can become oversaturated in the body, and it *is* possible to take too much—so periodic testing is a good idea if you're supplementing regularly. Too much vitamin D can lead to a buildup of calcium which can lead to other problems in the body.

CREATINE MONOHYDRATE

Creatine monohydrate is one of the most studied and widely used dietary supplements consistently proven to enhance exercise and athletic performance. Many people associate creatine exclusively with bodybuilding or strength training, but its benefits extend far beyond muscle building, particularly when it comes to brain health.

Creatine is naturally produced within your body and obtained from your diet in small amounts, primarily from animal products like meat. At the cellular level, it helps generate ATP (there it is again) by providing a phosphate group as a donor. To be clear, although you do absorb some from your diet, it would be extremely difficult to obtain optimal levels of creatine through diet alone—you would need to consume an unsafe (and comically large) amount of red meat to reach the recommended daily dose. Given what we've covered on nutrition, I don't recommend doing that.

Multiple studies conducted in both laboratory and active sports settings have found that creatine supplementation can significantly increase strength and power in both men and women. It has been shown to enhance muscle fiber recruitment for maximal effort contractions and improve overall athletic performance.

What's particularly interesting from a brain health perspective is that creatine can cross the blood-brain barrier via a protein called the creatine transporter (CRT). By allowing more creatine to enter the brain, this has been demonstrated to enhance cognitive performance and memory. Creatine has also been shown to have antioxidant properties in the brain, which can help protect neurons from toxicity, reduce mental fatigue, and potentially improve certain facets of neuropsychiatric disorders such as depression and bipolar disorder.

There is also emerging data showing enhanced recovery in traumatic brain injury patients, especially at higher doses, and even preliminary evidence suggesting creatine may serve as a possible preventive strategy for Alzheimer's and other forms of dementia.

While there is little data on whether creatine definitively impacts all-cause mortality, its known mechanisms and highly favorable safety profile make it a worthwhile supplement to consider. Even if it doesn't directly extend lifespan—although I wouldn't be surprised if we see data on this in the coming years—it's safe to say that it can certainly enhance your healthspan by providing improvements in strength and cognitive performance at the least.

Multiple studies have found virtually no consistent side effects from creatine use, except for potential weight gain due to increased water retention within muscles and increased muscle protein synthesis. That said, this weight gain tends to be a desired effect for many people looking to increase muscle mass and strength—and is not problematic in the same way that gaining weight (i.e., increasing fat stores) in other ways would be due to how metabolically active muscle is.

The current generally recommended dose of creatine monohydrate is 5–10 grams daily, although studies are underway to investigate the safety and efficacy of higher doses for longer-term use.

OMEGA-3 FATTY ACIDS (FISH OIL)

Fish oil is a common supplement that supplies a critical polyunsaturated fatty acid (PUFA) called omega-3, of which most Americans are deficient. According to a 2021 study analyzing NHANES data, approximately two-thirds of US adults and 95 percent of US children do not receive adequate omega-3s in their diet.

Within the omega-3 category, there are three main types: **DHA** (docosahexaenoic acid), **EPA** (eicosapentaenoic acid), and **ALA** (alpha-linolenic acid). DHA and EPA come from marine sources such as fish, whereas ALA is derived from plants. This distinction is important when selecting an omega-3 supplement as the quantities of DHA and EPA can vary dramatically from brand to brand, and getting the right amount of each is critical.

In multiple trials, DHA and EPA have been correlated with a reduction in all-cause mortality and appear to confer some longevity benefits. While ALA has been shown to provide similar effects, the data for DHA and EPA appears much stronger. For those interested, ALA is technically a precursor to EPA and DHA, but the conversion rate in the human body is relatively low, making it a less efficient source. If you follow a vegan or vegetarian diet for ethical reasons, it might be worth considering a marine-based omega-3 supplement despite your dietary choices, as the health benefits are significant.

A deficiency in omega-3s has been linked to a variety of cardiovascular diseases, while consistent use of omega-3 supplements has been correlated with improvements in memory and reduced risk of dementia, particularly Alzheimer's. This is not terribly surprising considering the fact that DHA makes up roughly 40 percent of all the fatty acids in your brain and is therefore crucial to your optimal brain function. Remember that your brain is also approximately 60 percent fat, so obtaining adequate amounts of these essential fatty acids is key for maintaining and optimizing your cognitive function.

Adequate supplementation has been correlated with a 17–21 percent reduction in all-cause mortality, which is among the highest of any supplement we'll discuss. Side effects can include minor gastrointestinal symptoms, a fishy aftertaste, and rarely, heart rhythm and skin issues.

The generally recommended daily intake is 500–1,000mg of DHA and 1,000–1,600mg of EPA, although there is evidence that up to 4,000mg daily (2,000mg of each form) is safe and effective in a dose-dependent fashion.

When selecting fish oil supplements, the quality here makes a big difference. Look for products that have been molecularly distilled to remove contaminants like heavy metals and PCBs. Products should also specify the exact amounts of DHA and EPA per serving, not just the total amount of fish oil. Third-party testing is also particularly important for fish oil supplements due to potential contamination issues. All this to say, it is worth doing your research here and potentially spending some extra money to take a high-quality fish oil at the correct dose.

CURCUMIN (TURMERIC)

Curcumin is the main active compound in turmeric, a spice made from the roots and rhizomes of the *Curcuma longa* plant. In multiple studies, it has been shown to postpone age-related changes in the body through several mechanisms. Curcumin lowers oxidative stress and inflammation, preserves telomere length, and impacts crucial signaling pathways for longevity. It has also been shown to upregulate AMPK and downregulate mTOR, which, as we've discussed, is beneficial for most people.

One challenge with curcumin is its relatively low bioavailability. Because it's isolated from a root and typically consumed as a powder, it can be difficult for your body to absorb. This is particularly true if you're simply using turmeric as a spice in cooking. Curcumin is fat-soluble, so it's more bioavailable when consumed with oils or when purchased in a gel form containing medium-chain triglyceride (MCT) or similar oil.

In multiple studies, curcumin appears to be safe with minimal to no side effects other than mild gastrointestinal symptoms. It's generally well-tolerated and has demonstrated up to a 10 percent reduction in all-cause mortality. It should be noted that it's also now widely available in capsule form, so you don't need to start adding turmeric to everything you cook! Although in my opinion it provides great flavor.

A daily dose of 500–1,000mg appears safe and likely confers many of the aforementioned benefits.

VITAMIN B12

Vitamin B12 is a water-soluble vitamin naturally present in certain foods such as eggs, milk, nutritional yeast, fish, and beef. It is required for the development, myelination, and overall function of your central nervous system. It's also crucial for healthy red blood cell formation and DNA synthesis, which makes it very important for your overall health. It's estimated that between 4–14 percent of US adults are deficient in vitamin B12.

Optimal levels of B12, along with B9 (folate) and B6, are linked with reduced cognitive decline in older adults. As you saw from Peter's story in the opening of this chapter, B12 deficiency can result in a reversible cause of dementia—meaning that if we correct the deficiency, we can often restore cognitive function that appeared to otherwise be lost. It's one of the critical tests neurologists run before labeling someone with Alzheimer's or other forms of dementia.

B12 also breaks down a compound called *homocysteine*. Observational studies have shown a positive association between elevated levels of homocysteine and the incidence of both Alzheimer's disease and other types of dementia. Elevated homocysteine levels may have negative effects on the brain through several mechanisms including impaired blood flow, deposition of tau protein (characteristic of Alzheimer's and TBI, as you may recall), and inhibition of methylation reactions—all of which can lead to neuroinflammation and ultimately accelerate brain aging through the premature death of more neurons.

Data on B12's impact on all-cause mortality is somewhat mixed. Low levels certainly increase mortality risk, but interestingly, elevated levels above the normal range also appear to increase this risk, as well. Therefore, maintaining B12 within the normal range seems to be the optimal approach, which can be easily assessed with bloodwork.

The recommended daily intake is quite low at just 2.4mcg, which can be achieved through diet or supplementation. For those who cannot absorb B12 properly through the digestive tract (a condition called pernicious anemia), sublingual supplements that dissolve under the tongue or even B12 injections may be necessary.

SPERMIDINE

Despite its unusual name (derived from its original discovery in semen, though it's found in many foods), spermidine is a natural polyamine found in wheat germ, whole grains, and various other foods. It has been shown to modulate aging, suppress the occurrence and severity of age-related diseases, and potentially prolong lifespan.

Autophagy—the cellular "recycling" process we've discussed in previous chapters—is thought to be the main mechanism through which spermidine delays aging and potentially extends lifespan. Studies have demonstrated improved autophagy in the liver, heart, and muscle tissues of mice, as well as delayed aging in yeast, worms, flies, and cultured mammalian cells. Spermidine also appears to lower inflammation, act as an antioxidant, improve proteostasis, regulate epigenetic factors, enhance lipid metabolism, and modulate cell growth and signaling pathways. That's checking multiple boxes from our hallmarks of aging!

Epidemiological data also suggests that increased dietary intake of spermidine may alleviate, delay, or halt specific age-dependent processes including cancer, cardiovascular disease, and dementia. Overall, the quality of data is not as robust in humans as with the previous examples but may still be worth considering. While there are no official recommendations for dosing, 5–15 mg per day appears safe and may be effective at activating some of these beneficial mechanisms.

NAD+ PRECURSORS

NAD+ (nicotinamide adenine dinucleotide) is a major coenzyme in your body that is central to mitochondrial function and the production of ATP. Without the production of either of these molecules, you would die within seconds. If you recall from Chapter 4, this is how cyanide works: it stops production of ATP in your mitochondria which kills you in a matter of minutes.

Lowered NAD+ levels in the body are associated with decreased energy production in the mitochondria, increased oxidative stress, DNA damage, cognitive impairment, and chronic inflammation. As we age, our NAD+ levels naturally decline, which has led researchers to investigate whether boosting these levels might slow or even reverse some aspects of aging.

There are two main precursors to NAD+ that have gained recent attention in the longevity space: **NMN (nicotinamide mononucleotide)** and **NR (nicotinamide riboside)**. While I could go into some of the science behind each of these and how they work, all you really need to know is that you can take both in supplement form and after ingestion, your body is then able to convert them into NAD+, which is why they're referred to as "precursors."

Technically speaking, there are other compounds like Niacin (vitamin B3) that can also be converted into NAD+. However, NMN and NR are considered closer to NAD+ and therefore require fewer steps to be converted, which is largely why they are now being explored as potential ways to increase NAD+ levels in the body.

Most of the research on these compounds has been conducted in animals, with human studies still in progress. The debate in the scientific community about their efficacy continues, with some researchers extremely optimistic about their potential while others remain skeptical until more human data is available. Neither compound appears to have significant safety concerns based on current research.

If you're interested in increasing NAD+ levels in your body, these supplements could be worth exploring. However, it's worth noting there are also well-established methods to increase your NAD+ levels that don't require supplements. These include calorie restriction, fasting, maintaining low overall glucose levels in the body, and regular exercise—all strategies we've already discussed.

Lastly, there are NAD+ infusions that can be given intravenously, but these can be costly and are generally described as unpleasant. Some people swear by them, but consider yourself warned.

POLYPHENOLS

Our final supplement worth mentioning is a category of compounds called polyphenols, which we've already touched on in a few places. These are generally found in the diet rather than taken as distinct supplements, but they serve as powerful antioxidants that can reduce oxidative stress, inflammation, and premature aging in the body. Polyphenols can impact specific hallmarks of aging such as cellular senescence and autophagy. They can also lower mTOR activity, boost sirtuin activation, assist with epigenetic regulation, and serve as mild hormetic stressors—a concept we explored in Chapter 8. While their overall impact remains somewhat unclear, they appear to increase lifespan by reducing the risk of many age-related chronic diseases we've already covered, such as cardiovascular disease, neurodegenerative disease, and metabolic issues like diabetes.

Dietary sources of polyphenols are abundant and include a variety of brightly colored vegetables, blueberries, blackberries, red onions, strawberries, olive oil, apples, nuts, grains, seeds, cloves, green and black tea, cocoa, coffee, and many others. Rather than taking a specific polyphenol supplement, focusing on incorporating these foods into your diet is likely the most effective strategy.

Personally, I consume about a tablespoon of olive oil every day for its high polyphenol count and the previously mentioned impacts on brain health. As mentioned in the Nutrition chapter, if you're looking to get some of your polyphenols from olive oil it's important to look for high-quality first cold press organic olive oil and consume it fresh.

YOUR SUPPLEMENT STRATEGY

As we reach the end of our brief exploration into supplements, it may surprise you to see how short this list is. There are many products we didn't cover here, many of which you've likely heard are beneficial and some of which you may take or have taken. To reiterate, I have chosen to focus on those that appear to have the best available human data on improving your longevity (except perhaps the NAD+ boosters, which remain contentious—I just felt the need to include them because of how often I see or hear about them). This does not mean there aren't others that may turn out to be as effective or even better; however, and I do my best to stay up on emerging data.

While I've presented some of the current evidence behind these supplements, I feel the need to say that I'm not suggesting you rush out and purchase any or every one of them. Everyone's individual needs will vary, and as we continue to gain more evidence, this list may well change. If you're interested in staying up to date on this kind of stuff, you can sign up for our newsletter at TranscendHealthGroup.com where we frequently send out updates on new studies and evidence-based health information. You can also download the full list of supplements with dosages on the book resource page, at TranscendHealthGroup.com/Resources, which we do update periodically.

One final step to consider before implementing any new supplement is to have appropriate bloodwork done to assess your levels if applicable. Your primary care doctor may be able to perform some of this basic bloodwork, but I would suggest looking into more comprehensive tests, many of which are now commercially available without a prescription. There are many services now offering this and that are able to provide personalized recommendations for proper supplementation. The doses mentioned here are merely general benchmarks—optimal ranges can vary between individuals based on diet, body mass index, genetic factors, and other variables. So, if you do regularly take supplements, it would be worth monitoring your bloodwork on a routine basis, typically quarterly.

Remember that supplements are *supplementary* to a healthy lifestyle. Far and away, the best things you can do for your brain, body, and overall longevity are to focus on consistent exercise, proper nutrition, effective stress management, and getting enough high-quality sleep. That's not to say you should ignore supplements but that, generally speaking, taking a pill without adhering to the first four pillars is not going to drastically change your life. Consistently doing all the above, however, just might.

KEY TAKEAWAYS

1. **Supplements should complement the fundamentals, not replace them.** Supplements are supplementary by nature and can enhance the benefits of proper exercise, nutrition, stress management, and sleep—but they are not a substitute for them. Within a comprehensive longevity framework, they're best viewed as an addition, offering targeted support for specific health needs rather than miracle solutions. Given the relative ease of implementation, there aren't many downsides to taking them as long as they are needed.

2. **Most people have nutritional gaps despite adequate nutrition.** Approximately half of the US population and more than two billion people worldwide are deficient in at least one micronutrient. Modern food production methods, lifestyle factors, and environmental conditions make it challenging to obtain optimal nutrition from diet alone. Targeted supplementation can help address these common deficiencies.

3. **Micronutrient deficiencies can cause damage well before symptoms appear.** Your body can compensate for nutritional deficiencies for years before noticeable symptoms develop. By the time clinical signs emerge, underlying mechanisms may have already accelerated the aging process or contributed to disease development. Regular testing and appropriate supplementation can address these deficiencies long before they cause damage that can't be easily reversed.

You can find a list of all the specific interventions from this chapter in the Supplements Cheat Sheet at TranscendHealthGroup.com/Resources.

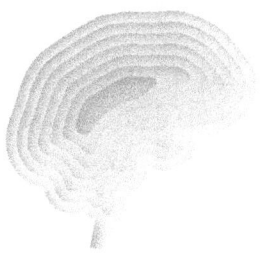

CHAPTER 10
TECHNOLOGY

JAMES SOFTLY AWAKENS as the gentle hum of his bedroom shades begins their programmed morning ascent. A warm amber glow filters through the windows, bathing his face in the early dawn light. He blinks away the remnants of sleep, feeling that familiar clarity and lightness in his body—a sensation he hasn't taken for granted since his late forties, when mornings used to mean stiff joints and brain fog. Now, at fifty-seven, he springs out of bed with the energy of someone half his age.

"Good morning, James," comes a pleasant voice from the doorway. It's Hermes, his household humanoid robot, carrying a tray with freshly ground coffee and a small arrangement of pills and capsules—his personalized supplement regimen. "You achieved an impressive eight hours and ten minutes of sleep last night, with excellent REM and deep sleep cycles. Your recovery metrics are optimal today."

James sits up, accepting the coffee with a grateful nod. "Thanks, Hermes."

"The temperature outside is 54°," Hermes continues, "so you might want a light jacket for Buck and Heidi's morning walk—unless you're planning on some more intentional cold exposure. Your stress biomarkers indicate you'd handle it well today."

As James slips on his smart glasses, the data Hermes mentioned materializes in his field of view, confirming his biometric data from overnight: sleep cycles, heart rate variability, body temperature, blood pressure—all within ideal ranges. He remembers when those numbers first started improving five years ago and smiles to himself knowing how far he has come since then. Global headlines scroll discretely across his periphery as he makes his way downstairs, his movements fluid and confident.

"Good morning, James," comes another voice—this one from his home system speakers. "I see you've taken your morning supplements. I hope you're enjoying the new Colombian blend—I made sure Hermes prepared it to your preferences. Your exercise regimen today calls for forty-five minutes of steady-state cardio. I've prepared your stationary bike with a fresh towel and water bottle. Your quarterly mobile blood draw is scheduled for 9:00 a.m., and you have a meeting with Bill from Stark, Inc. at 11 a.m. to discuss your collaboration. Breakfast will be ready when you return from your walk. Your schedule should permit a twenty-minute stop at the park, if you'd like. Buck and Heidi would also benefit from their cardiovascular exercise."

James reaches for his dogs' leashes and smiles as they come bounding up to him. At ten and eleven years old, they still have the energy and playfulness of puppies. He feels a surge of gratitude knowing he's giving them the best life possible and that he'll have them in his life for well past their previously expected age range.

Just five years ago, this morning would have seemed like something from a science fiction novel. Now, it's just another Tuesday—and there are many, many more to come.

CURRENT TECHNOLOGY

If this sounds like science fiction, you might be surprised to learn that every piece of technology described in James's morning routine exists today. While most of us don't experience this level of integration, it's only a matter of time before some version of this becomes commonplace for all of us. And this doesn't even begin to account for technologies still under development or those yet to be invented. In fact, by the time this book gets in your hands there will be even more extreme examples of technological change, because it's happening that fast.

Therefore, given the accelerating rate of technological advancement, it's nearly impossible to predict what our lives might look like in five, ten, or twenty years. One thing is certain, however: if we harness and implement these developments correctly, they have enormous potential to extend human healthspan and lifespan. And many of them are already here.

In this chapter, we'll review how current technologies may fit into your longevity framework and take a look at what might be coming in the near future. While I highly doubt any emerging technology will replace or invalidate the fundamentals we've already covered, there is little doubt that technology is going to be an increasingly large part of the longevity puzzle and only serve to enhance an integrated, healthy lifestyle.

With that in mind, I'd like to start with what's available today. Perhaps the most accessible and immediately useful technology for longevity is continuous health monitoring through wearable devices. If you're reading this book, there's a good chance you already have or are at least aware of one of these devices. If not, you may be ready to purchase one by the end.

WEARABLE DEVICES

There are already a variety of devices on the market today that can track your physiologic data in real time. In no particular order, popular options include:

- Apple Watch
- Whoop Band
- Oura Ring
- Samsung Galaxy Watch
- Fitbit Sense
- Amazfit GTR

While these devices vary in their specifics, most track similar metrics that directly correlate to your current health and overall longevity. These aren't just novelties—they provide actionable, real-time data about the function of your various organ systems that were previously only available through specialized medical equipment. I still marvel at the fact that what has classically taken a room full of hospital equipment can now sit on your finger or wrist, reminiscent of the original ENIAC computer compared to a modern-day laptop. Of course, the information these devices provide is only one part of the puzzle. You can have all the data in the world, but if you don't do anything with it, it likely won't do you much good.

Therefore, to make a wearable device useful, you need to first understand what information it tracks, how to analyze it, and then how to integrate actionable changes into your life. Let's take a look at some of the most important metrics these devices provide and what they might mean for your own longevity framework.

SLEEP QUALITY AND DURATION

We already know that consistently achieving an adequate duration of high-quality sleep is one of the best longevity interventions at your disposal. But sleep is a difficult metric to track on your own—you typically don't know exactly when you fall asleep or wake up to the minute, and relying on your personal recollection to understand the quality of your sleep is essentially impossible.

Modern wearable devices are extremely useful for tracking not just how long you sleep but can also provide a rudimentary assessment of your sleep stages (light, deep, and REM), and your sleep efficiency. By now, you're already well aware that seven to nine hours are optimal for most adults. However, it's worth noting that longer sleep durations have also been associated with increased all-cause mortality: as much as 27 percent for anything beyond nine hours, 53 percent for ten hours or more, and up to 84 percent for eleven hours of sleep on average.

In Chapter 7, we also discussed the importance of sleep consistency. A 2024 study published in the journal *Sleep* examined 1,859 people over nearly eight years and found that higher sleep regularity was associated with a 20–48 percent lower all-cause mortality, a 16–39 percent lower cancer mortality, and a 22–57 percent lower cardiovascular disease mortality. This highlights the importance of maintaining a consistent sleep schedule, which is something many wearable devices can help you achieve.

To be clear, the best method we currently have for truly knowing which sleep stage you are in is a polysomnogram, or a dedicated sleep study, which we also referenced in Chapter 7. This involves another complex array of equipment including an electroencephalogram (EEG) to measure your brain wave activity, an electromyogram (EMG) to measure muscle activity, an electrooculogram (EOG) to measure eye movement, and an EKG to measure heart activity. It also measures parameters like pulse oximetry, respiratory rate and pattern, and records a live video to help detect movement and breathing patterns. This currently requires referral to a sleep laboratory to complete, but it takes no stretch of the imagination to conceptualize that this will likely be available at home in the near future for those who require this level of assessment.

The point is that our current wearable technologies provide a basic overview of some of these data points, but they are still not as precise as a full-blown sleep study. Therefore, I would not live and die by the information they present but rather use them as a relative gauge to observe trends in your body after changing a particular behavior and using that feedback to adjust your habits accordingly.

As a personal example, after limiting my alcohol intake to near zero over the past several years (especially closer to bedtime), I have observed and felt the quality of my sleep markedly improve. As a painful reminder to myself, after enjoying a couple glasses of Caymus cabernet on my birthday this year, I was gifted a poor night's sleep with data that supported it, and an unrestful start to my new year. I assure you I am still learning with you.

RESTING HEART RATE

Your resting heart rate is another surprisingly powerful predictor of your longevity, and something that nearly every wearable device can easily track. A 2013 Mayo Clinic study of over 53,000 patients found that individuals with a resting heart rate below 60 BPM had a 38–66 percent lower all-cause mortality than individuals with a resting heart rate above 80 BPM. This correlation remained even after adjusting for factors like BMI, smoking, alcohol use, and physical activity.

Another 2013 publication in the journal *Heart* followed 2,798 Danish men for sixteen years and found a 16 percent increased risk of all-cause mortality for every additional ten-beat increase in resting heart rate. If you use a wearable device, you should be able to not only monitor your heart rate in real time but also analyze trends over time. Consistent exercise, proper nutrition, quality sleep, and effectively managing stress are all excellent ways to lower your resting heart rate. Any of these sound familiar? If you choose to implement any of the interventions in this book, one possible way to judge their efficacy would be to look at your resting heart rate—which, in theory, should start trending downward.

For most healthy adults, a resting heart rate between 50–70 BPM is considered optimal. Athletes may achieve even lower rates, sometimes in the 30 or 40s, which is typically a sign of excellent cardiovascular conditioning. While extremely low heart rates for a non-athlete (below 40 BPM) can be concerning, a gradual decrease in resting heart rate as you implement the various types of exercise from Chapter 5 is a generally positive sign.

HEART RATE VARIABILITY (HRV)

HRV measures the variation in time between each heartbeat, typically represented in milliseconds. Higher variability generally indicates better cardiovascular health and greater resilience to stress as it is an indirect indicator of higher parasympathetic tone—meaning more time in the "rest and digest" state and less in "fight or flight" mode. Therefore, a higher HRV number is better than a lower number. In fact, a 2022 meta-analysis looking at thirty-two studies with over 38,000 participants in total demonstrated a 56 percent increase in all-cause mortality in individuals in the lowest quartile of HRV compared to all other quartiles.

Additionally a 2024 twin study published in the *Journal of the American Heart Association* examined over 500 individuals and showed a 22 percent lower risk of all-cause mortality in those with higher HRV suggesting the relevance of this metric despite identical genetics.

HRV also varies significantly from person to person and naturally decreases with age. For example, a healthy HRV range for a thirty-to-thirty-nine-year-old male might be between 45–85ms, while for someone over seventy years, it might be between 10–45ms. Rather than focusing on absolute values, what's likely more relevant is tracking your personal trends over time. As you continue to implement healthy lifestyle changes, you should expect to see your HRV trend upward.

BODY TEMPERATURE

Normal body temperature typically ranges from 97.8–99°F (36.5–37.2°C). While minor fluctuations are normal, consistently elevated temperatures may indicate inflammation or infection, both of which can contribute to accelerated aging.

Tracking your temperature trends over time can help you identify patterns and potential health issues before they become serious. Wearables can track your body temperature, including natural fluctuations throughout the day and night, which as we previously discussed are also an indicator of quality sleep as your core temperature drops overnight before it rises again the closer you are to waking. These measurements can also help detect early signs of illness, as elevated temperatures often precede other symptoms, and can help with family planning by tracking monthly temperature fluctuations, which correlate with female ovulation.

RESPIRATORY RATE

Your respiratory rate—the number of breaths you take per minute—is another vital sign that can correlate with your overall health. For healthy adults at rest, a normal respiratory rate typically ranges from twelve to twenty breaths per minute. Lower rates generally indicate better cardiovascular efficiency, while consistently elevated rates may suggest underlying respiratory issues or heightened stress.

For context, a 2022 study of 853 patients aged sixty or older found approximately a 14 percent increased risk of all-cause mortality for each additional breath per minute increase in their respiratory rate.

Like resting heart rate, your respiratory rate should gradually decrease as you become more physically fit. This is a positive trend that suggests your body is becoming more efficient at oxygen utilization. Most wearable devices can calculate your estimated respiratory rate based on your heart rate, which tends to be fairly accurate.

OXYGEN SATURATION

Oxygen saturation (often represented as SpO2) measures the percentage of hemoglobin in your blood that is carrying oxygen. Normal levels typically range from 95–100 percent. Consistently low oxygen saturation (below 90 percent) can indicate respiratory or cardiovascular issues that require medical attention. For instance, a 2024 study in the *Journal of Clinical Sleep Medicine* examined over 4,800 adults over a period of eleven years and found that nighttime oxygen saturation levels below 94 percent were associated with progressively increased mortality risk, while each 1 percent increase above 95 percent corresponded to a 7 percent decreased risk of all-cause mortality.

While minor fluctuations are normal, particularly during sleep, your oxygen saturation should generally remain above 95 percent during waking hours. Tracking this metric can be particularly valuable for those with respiratory conditions or who live at high altitudes. A drop in oxygen saturation can also indicate an infection, especially a pneumonia, as the ability to exchange oxygen across the lungs is diminished and the body's metabolic demands increase in response to fighting an infection.

PHYSICAL ACTIVITY

Most wearable devices also track various aspects of physical activity, including steps taken, distance traveled, calories burned, and time spent being active. While these metrics are not direct indicators of your health like the previously mentioned vital signs, they can be incredibly valuable. This type of information can provide motivation, accountability, and help you make better decisions about your health by reviewing trends over time.

The general goal, of course, should be to maintain consistent levels of physical activity as you age. You can consult the cheat sheet from Chapter 5 for more details around exactly how much exercise to shoot for on a weekly basis, although most wearable devices have software that will simply tell you whether or not you're achieving enough. Those recommendations are likely a good place to start, and over time you can review your trends and make sure you're hitting the required targets for your goals.

This is one way that you can use technology to "gamify" your health. Devices like the Apple Watch, for example, can encourage you to meet your daily targets for physical activity by "filling your rings" and even allow you to compete with your friends in week-long physical challenges. It might sound silly, but turning exercise into a fun type of game, or doing so in a group setting by sharing with friends, have both been shown to be helpful.

Remember that wearable devices can only provide so much information. At the time of writing this, most wearables are essentially conducting daily checks on your vital signs. That said, maintaining these vital signs within optimal ranges has been well correlated with an increased longevity in large populations of people studied.

While all these metrics are valuable, I would argue that based upon currently available evidence, optimizing your heart rate, HRV, and metrics around your physical activity are particularly among the most powerful to track.

DIAGNOSTICS

So, how can you obtain data on all the things that wearable devices *can't* measure? This is where laboratory testing and advanced diagnostics come in. These deeper assessments complement wearable device data to create a more comprehensive picture of your health status and overall longevity trajectory.

One of the best ways to obtain a more comprehensive look at your overall health is through bloodwork. Unfortunately, annual bloodwork from your primary care doctor likely isn't thorough or frequent enough in tracking many of the longevity markers we now know to look for. As we've discussed, the traditional Western healthcare system isn't incentivized to focus on prevention, which often leads to inadequate testing that may miss subtle yet important markers of accelerated aging or disease risk.

For those serious about their longevity, more frequent and comprehensive testing provides insights that wearables simply cannot detect.

There are a handful of subscription services now available that allow you to check many if not all the following biomarkers at a reasonable cost. If you're wanting to keep an eye on these, quarterly testing is fairly ideal as it provides enough time to meaningfully change habits and see results reflected on the following set. More often may not provide enough time to see changes—not to mention is costly and time consuming—and waiting longer may miss opportunities to correct course sooner. Many common biomarkers to consider include:

- **Complete Blood Count (CBC):** A measure of your red and white blood cells and platelets, providing insight into your immune function, oxygen-carrying capacity, and overall health.
- **C-Reactive Protein (CRP) and high-sensitivity CRP (hs-CRP):** Markers of inflammation in your body, with lower levels generally indicating better health and longevity.
- **Apolipoprotein-B (ApoB):** Measures a structural component that helps transport fats and cholesterol in the bloodstream and is a stronger predictor of cardiovascular risk than standard cholesterol measurements.
- **Lipoprotein(a):** A genetic variant of LDL cholesterol that significantly increases cardiovascular risk independent of other risk factors known to affect up to 25 percent of people worldwide.
- **Cholesterol and triglycerides:** Measure the amount of fats and ratio of lipids in the bloodstream, which can also be helpful to stratify cardiovascular disease risk.
- **Hemoglobin A1c (HbA1c):** Reflects your average blood glucose over approximately three months, giving a longer-term picture of metabolic health than spot glucose readings.
- **Fasting insulin:** Measures the hormone that regulates blood sugar, with lower values generally indicating better insulin sensitivity and metabolic health.

- **Basic metabolic panel:** Assesses your overall electrolyte balance, kidney function, and basics of your acid-base balance and metabolic function.
- **Liver function tests (AST, ALT, GGT):** Enzymes indicating how well your liver is functioning, which is an organ crucial for detoxification and metabolic health.
- **Creatine kinase:** Helps monitor muscle breakdown and recovery and can be particularly important for those engaging in regular exercise.
- **Vitamin D:** Critical for bone health, immune function, and numerous cellular processes throughout the body.
- **8-OHdG (8-hydroxy-2'-deoxyguanosine):** Indicates the level of DNA damage from oxidative stress, with lower levels suggesting better cellular health.
- **Hormone panel (testosterone, SHBG, estradiol, progesterone, cortisol):** Provide insight into your endocrine system, which affects everything from energy to mood to tissue repair.
- **Cortisol:** Measures the level of this particular stress hormone in the blood, which can correlate to overall adrenal function and sympathetic tone.
- **B12/folate:** Measures levels of each in the bloodstream, which can be predictive of risk for certain types of anemia and neurologic disorders like memory loss.
- **Ferritin and iron panel:** Measures overall iron stores in the body and circulating iron in the bloodstream, which is necessary for red blood cell formation and overall inflammation.
- **TSH/T3/T4:** Measures levels of thyroid hormones in the bloodstream, which are a reflection of an over- or underactive thyroid.
- **The Galleri Test:** A cutting-edge blood test that is capable of detecting multiple cancer types before symptoms appear by identifying DNA shed from tumor cells in the bloodstream.

- **Gut microbiome analysis:** Tests like Viome (which is a stool, not blood test) analyze your gut microbiome composition, which influences immune function, inflammation, and even brain health.
- **DNA methylation:** Tests like TruMe (which is a cheek swab, not blood test) and others analyze the methylation patterns of your DNA, which are known to influence gene expression and can provide a representation of your rate of cellular or biological aging.

IMAGING

Medical imaging refers to technology that is used to create visual representations of the interior of the body, which you can then use to gain health insights and diagnose potential problems without invasive surgical procedures. You're probably already aware of common imaging tools like X-rays and MRIs. Imaging technologies are typically used when things go wrong, but like many aspects of Western medicine, we may be ignoring their use as a form of preventive medicine.

While the data around the necessity of regular imaging is somewhat mixed, these technologies are now developing as another useful tool in our longevity arsenal. They're also improving quickly and becoming more universally available.

For our purposes, there are a few types of imaging that are at least worth knowing about as you build your own longevity framework and may be worth looking into depending on your goals or unique situation.

CLEERLY CT

In Chapter 3, we briefly touched on the Cleerly CT scan, which is a sophisticated imaging tool that provides a detailed picture of the coronary vessels in the heart. With assistance from AI, it can reliably determine the characteristics of arterial plaques and identify the likelihood of a blockage occurring that may result in a heart attack before it happens. This can allow for a planned intervention to deploy a stent, repair a vessel, or even change your lifestyle or medication regimen before a potentially fatal event.

Unlike traditional coronary calcium scoring, which primarily identifies calcified (hard) plaque, Cleerly CT technology actually distinguishes between soft and hard plaque within the coronary vessels. This distinction is important because soft plaque is significantly more vulnerable to rupture, which can trigger a heart attack. Traditional calcium scoring might miss these dangerous soft plaques entirely, giving patients a false sense of security despite carrying significant cardiovascular risk.

To put it simply, this is a pretty incredible technology. Never before in human history have we been able to predict an individual's likelihood of heart attack with this level of accuracy. As such, the Cleerly CT can be a powerful tool for patients with family histories of heart disease or other risk factors. That said, this is not something that should stand alone as a means to weigh your risk and otherwise throw caution to the wind. Improving your cardiovascular health through the fundamental interventions we've already covered is among the best known ways to effectively do so.

WHOLE-BODY MRI

Commercial whole-body MRI has emerged as one of the most comprehensive screening tools available today. Unlike traditional MRIs that focus on specific anatomic regions, whole-body MRI scans can provide a complete picture of your entire body in a single session. This technology allows for the detection of abnormalities across multiple organ systems without exposure to ionizing radiation, making it a safer alternative to CT scans for regular screening.

The benefits of whole-body MRI include early detection of various conditions such as tumors, vascular abnormalities, and inflammatory diseases before they manifest as symptoms. There is an argument that MRIs may lead to overdiagnosis and false positive findings that result in unnecessary procedures and interventions. I am personally of the opinion that I would rather have more information at my disposal to make an informed decision rather than finding out too late that I could have done something about a problem much sooner. For a more sobering example, nearly half of all cancers are diagnosed at stage III or IV, where survival rates are far lower than when they are discovered at stages I or II. Either way, this is a personal decision.

DEXA SCAN

Similarly, a DEXA scan (dual energy X-ray absorptiometry) is considered the gold standard for monitoring bone mineral density and is therefore useful in detecting osteopenia or osteoporosis. This has massive implications with respect to fracture risk after sustaining an injury or fall, which can impact all-cause mortality in our later years.

Beyond bone health, DEXA scans can also measure your ratio of lean body mass to fat mass, which is predictive of your metabolic health. These can provide far more insights than simple weight measurements or BMI calculations, like determining your level of muscle compared to visceral fat for example.

DEXA scans can also help guide the effectiveness of a treatment regimen to see how your body responds to certain interventions like exercise training programs, vitamin D supplementation, and more. It's also worth noting that the amount of radiation from a DEXA scan is incredibly low, far less than a standard X-ray, so frequency is much less of a concern.

To reiterate, medical imaging is advancing rapidly, in large part due to advancements in AI. This rapidly evolving technology is able to detect patterns and abnormalities that even the most highly trained doctors might miss, and even more critically, it can now detect markers that were previously unknown to us. This is all happening at an incredibly fast rate, which means the future of medical imaging—and medical technology in general—is incredibly hard to predict.

But let's have a little fun, shall we? Let's shift gears and consider some of the exciting technologies that might be coming down the pipeline, some sooner than you may think.

FUTURE TECHNOLOGY

While current technology offers powerful tools for monitoring and diagnosing an array of potential health issues, my prediction is that advancements in the next five, ten, and certainly even twenty years will make our current wearable devices look archaic. Some of these future technologies are almost inevitable—they're currently in their infancy or even being deployed in niche ways not yet available to the public—while others remain speculative. Either way, the future of longevity medicine and truly preventive health appears bright.

THE ARTIFICIAL DOCTOR WILL SEE YOU NOW

As I mentioned in Chapter 2, AI agents have already passed the MCAT, USMLE, and multiple medical specialty boards—including mine, the American Board of Psychiatry and Neurology. In the case of the latter, in December of 2024 it didn't just pass the exam, it performed *better* than the average neurologist. Therefore, the idea of an AI agent functioning as your personal physician is not at all far-fetched. In fact, I would say it is only a matter of time until this is reality, especially considering the already prevalent use of AI in medicine.

Neurologists, radiologists, and neurosurgeons have been using AI for almost the last decade to help save millions of lives and trillions of neurons. For example, Viz.ai, an app created in 2016, allows for AI-guided assistance to detect the presence of large vessel occlusions (blockages of major arteries in the brain) that can cause debilitating strokes. I have personally used this technology for years and can say that it absolutely enhances my judgment and improves patient outcomes, and this is just one of several iterations.

Treating emergent strokes is part of my day job, and that process involves looking at STAT brain vessel imaging for each patient that comes through the door. Viz often saves crucial time as I can simply take a second look at what it has found, compare it with my own assessment, briefly discuss it with an interventionist, and then send a given patient for a potentially brain-saving procedure often stops an active stroke in its tracks. This is just one application of this incredible technology, and it has no doubt saved countless lives and debility.

As another example of AI in healthcare, large language models are already trained on an array of preventive and functional medicine topics designed to help coach patients through a number of medical scenarios, which will only continue to improve. I suspect that it is only a matter of time before a medically trained AI agent is hooked up to a wearable device on your body, allowing it to perform digital examinations, interpret a live readout of your vital signs, and render an accurate diagnosis and treatment plan for whatever problems you may encounter in real time.

There are even companies training large language models on interpreting facial recognition to detect various disease processes with remarkable accuracy, making this scenario even more feasible over a simple video chat or call. For legal reasons, a provider will likely need to sign off on that decision before a given treatment is administered, but most of the heavy lifting will likely be done or at the very least augmented by these digital agents very soon.

I realize this might sound almost dystopian to some. There is certainly something to be said for working with a human being—their empathy and bedside manner can go a long way, especially in dealing with sensitive topics and life-changing diagnoses. But I would also argue that AI might eventually provide a better experience in this arena, as well. While I was fortunate to have excellent mentors who demonstrated compassionate care during my medical training and who I have done my best to emulate, I'm sure we've all encountered physicians who could use a refresher course in bedside manner.

Properly trained AI agents won't have this problem. They won't feel tired, hungry, sleep-deprived, or overworked. They won't be distracted by personal issues or conflicts with colleagues. They'll simply perform as programmed, with self-reinforcing behavior that continuously improves how they serve patients. It's a strange thought, but not at all a stretch of the imagination considering where we are today.

What's more, **artificial general intelligence (AGI)** might be closer than many of us realize too. The term AGI refers to the idea that artificial intelligence may eventually be able to replicate human-like intelligence, including emotional intelligence. Some experts believe this has already happened, while others estimate it's just decades away. With continuous self-learning and processing power far beyond what the human brain can achieve, AI could potentially combine the diagnostic brilliance of the most knowledgeable physicians with the empathy and communication skills of the most compassionate ones, resulting in far better patient outcomes and vastly improved healthcare for everyone.

Personally, I find this incredibly exciting—even as someone whose job might be on the line. While I'm not exactly fearful of losing my job to AI anytime soon, I'm certainly in favor of anything that will help save lives and improve the overall health of our population. If that means I have to hand my white coat over to a robot that's better than me in every way, so be it.

With that said, let's explore some of the more speculative technologies that may also be on the horizon. We'll start with the most likely and end with the most far-fetched.

NANOBOTS

Similar to artificial intelligence, nanobots represent a potential new frontier in medical technology. Nanobots are microscopic machines measured on a scale of nanometers (one billionth of a meter) that could potentially perform a variety of task within your body, such as:

- Real-time surveillance of blood composition
- Cellular repair
- Waste product removal
- Cancer cell destruction
- Targeted drug delivery

While nanotechnology is still an area of active development and research, some believe that we could see clinical applications of these devices as early as the 2030s. The implications of nanotechnology are potentially massive when we consider their impact on the hallmarks of aging and even the possibility of *reversing* cellular aging.

Imagine, for example, being able to reverse your DNA damage and lengthen your telomeres, which could improve the fidelity of your protein synthesis and overall function of your cells. Alternatively, if your proteins begin to malfunction and become misfolded and aggregate within different tissues in your body, nanobots could be on the lookout for these damaged molecules and sweep them away as necessary. They could even potentially detect things like abnormal markers on early cancer cells or pro-inflammatory cytokines secreted by senescent cells, then mark them for destruction before they have a chance to spread or impact local, healthy cells. The applications are nearly endless.

BRAIN-COMPUTER INTERFACES (BCIS)

A brain-computer interface (BCI) is a device that allows direct communication between the brain and an external device. The company Neuralink, founded by Elon Musk, has successfully implanted devices in at least three patients as of early 2025, and perhaps even more by the time you read this.

These devices can be implanted within the brain or spinal cord, which is just as sci-fi as it sounds. They are able to record electrical activity in your brain and nervous system which is then processed, transmitted to an external device, and decoded. Imagine thinking about the word "longevity" and then seeing it on your computer screen, without having to type it out. That's essentially what's happening—these devices can translate electrical impulses in your brain into something you can actually comprehend and use.

One phenomenal application for BCIs is to help people with disabilities. For example, a patient with quadriplegia could have the device implanted in their brain to record electrical activity as they think about moving. The device could then process these signals and wirelessly transmit them to a computer, allowing the patient to control digital interfaces using only their thoughts. This is precisely what happened with Noland Arbaugh, the first known patient to receive a Neuralink implant, who has famously played the Nintendo classic Mario Kart *with his mind.*

Several companies, including Synchron, Blackrock Neurotech, and Kernel, are developing similar technologies. While the initial applications focus on helping people overcome disabilities, the long-term potential extends far beyond that, potentially even to include superhuman abilities like telepathic communication or the ability to rapidly download external information.

The implications for how we learn, the framework of our formal education system, and even our roles in the workplace could all look completely different than what we know today. Like Neo in *The Matrix*, you too might one day utter the phrase, "I know Kung Fu."

AUGMENTED SENSORY DEVICES

An augmented sensory device is a technology that enhances or extends human sensory perception by providing additional information or altering existing sensory inputs, often through wearable or body-attached devices.

For example, most of us are familiar with corrective lenses like glasses or contact lenses that compensate for myopia (nearsightedness) or presbyopia (age-related farsightedness). These devices can help return our vision to normal, but what if there were a device that could enhance your vision beyond what the normal human visual apparatus is designed to see? This may be possible through augmented sensory devices—in the case of vision, something akin to a "bionic eye."

Consider the fact that humans can only see the "visible light spectrum," which we've appropriately named. The electromagnetic spectrum, however, is far broader than what our eyes can detect. For example, UV rays are not visible to us, but they are to honeybees. In fact, this is how they navigate to the center of a flower even on a cloudy day. The idea of expanding our vision through augmented sensory devices is not that far-fetched, and the possibilities are pretty wild. For the Superman fans out there, X-ray vision could give you the ability to see through walls. You could improve your night vision or perhaps even install a zoom feature, giving your eyes adjustable, telescopic vision. These are all possible scenarios that are currently being investigated with applications that range from the military battlefield to recreational.

Similar enhancements could also apply to hearing. Hearing aids and cochlear implants already help those with hearing loss, but future technology might enable hearing beyond the normal human range—perhaps as acute as a dog's hearing, which can detect sounds four times farther away and across a broader range of frequencies.

Exoskeletons are another type of augmented sensory device that are already being used to help patients with physical disabilities or neurologic injuries to walk or move again. But think about the endless potential applications of these devices—they could also be used to safely lift heavy objects outside the range of maximum human strength or reduce wear and tear on joints and connective tissue. And, of course, they could provide another tool to help us all stay active well into our old age.

These are all current and future possibilities that may allow you to augment your natural abilities, and this doesn't even include future technologies that haven't even been thought of or invented yet. It is not outside the realm of possibility to think that you may have the potential to become what we would think of as a superhero in the coming decades, with a combination of these devices working in tandem to augment your abilities and even repair your body in real time, keeping you younger and more vibrant for longer.

AND NOW, THE REALLY WEIRD

Beyond these relatively conceivable technologies lies another realm of possibilities that is almost impossible to wrap your head around. (There's our linear thinking, holding us back again.) Without getting into too many details, and because they aren't entirely known yet, here are some interesting scenarios that *might* be possible within your lifetime.

- **The singularity:** This term, recently popularized by futurist Ray Kurzweil, refers to a theoretical point at which technological growth becomes so uncontrollable and irreversible that it results in the merging of human consciousness and artificial intelligence. As dystopian as this sounds, Kurzweil's version is one that elevates the collective consciousness of humanity and grants us abilities and a reality far beyond our current frame of reference or conception. I'll let you ponder that at your own risk.
- **Longevity escape velocity:** This concept describes reaching a point in humanity where technology extends human lifespan by at least one year for every year we live, effectively rendering aging optional. Kurzweil also predicts this could happen between 2029

and 2035, while longevity researcher Aubrey de Grey suggests this will be a reality closer to the late 2030s. Others still believe this is only a theoretical possibility. Time will tell.
- **Digital consciousness:** Sometimes called "mind uploading," this refers to the theoretical possibility of transferring human consciousness to a digital format, potentially allowing a form of digital immortality.
- **Quantum computing and advancements in physics:** Breakthroughs in these fields could lead to technologies we can't even conceptualize within our current framework of understanding, with several of these computers already in production today solving equations at speeds we previously thought were impossible.

While these concepts might seem far-fetched, remember that many of today's commonplace technologies—smartphones, the internet, genetic sequencing—would have seemed equally impossible just a few generations ago, and the possibilities are only accelerating.

THE FUTURE OF LONGEVITY

Within the longevity space, there are really two main camps: those who put their faith in technology and those who put their faith in the fundamentals. Personally, I have a foot in each, although I currently lean more toward the fundamentals because that is what the evidence currently demonstrates to be true. However, I am hopeful and confident that technology will continue to radically inform and change the way we approach human longevity in the coming decades. As we just covered, it is very difficult to know exactly what that might look like or when those technologies may ultimately be accessible to everyone.

There is a very real possibility that aging becomes optional within your lifetime and that you'll be able to utilize technology to optimize your body in ways you can't even imagine today. But as exciting as that sounds, I don't think it's something you should count on quite yet.

The reality is that you have the power to significantly increase the health and performance of your brain and body *right now*, and largely without the need to rely on technology. The fundamental pillars of longevity—exercise, nutrition, stress management, and sleep—will always remain essential, and they will always get you far. Technology can and will likely continue to enhance these pillars in the future, but I am doubtful that it will ever fully replace them. As of now, I would assume that these fundamentals will remain an integral part of your optimal wellness strategy for the foreseeable future.

I believe the future of longevity will neither be shaped strictly by technology nor the fundamentals in isolation, but by a synergistic relationship between the two. Technology is a tool that can be used to extend our natural capabilities, amplify our efforts, and unlock new potentials we're only beginning to understand.

Technology is already used as a force multiplier for intentional living, and it's likely only going to get better. Right now, we have devices that track our vitals, apps that provide customized workout routines, and services that generate customized supplement regimens. Now imagine having an AI coach, like James, who doesn't just hand you a workout routine but creates a perfectly optimized exercise program tailored to your unique preferences, genetic predispositions, even your schedule. Furthermore, consider how continuous monitoring could be used to solve the age-old question of exactly which nutritional and pharmacologic approach works best for *your* body, not just what has been shown to work well for the general population.

There's a not-so-distant future where *your* decisions about *your* health aren't just informed by general principles, but by real-time feedback from devices that are able to learn more about the intricacies of your body than any doctor ever could. One where your treatments are prescribed and implemented in real time, long before the first symptom or preventable complication arises.

Personally, I don't see this diminishing the importance of our own knowledge base, but rather, enhancing it. Technology provides us with more and better tools, but we will still need the wisdom to implement them effectively. Even the most advanced innovations will only work best when paired with your self-awareness and conscious choice. Not to mention, a nanobot can't give you purpose, and a brain-computer interface can't manufacture the will to live well. An AI doctor can prescribe near-perfect interventions, but it can't make you care enough to follow through on them.

I'm most excited not about what these tools can do for us, but how they can free us up to focus on what truly matters. As the drudgery of routine health maintenance becomes increasingly automated, you'll be able to devote more of your time and energy to achieving your why. To *living life*. That's what this is all about.

You'll always have a choice. I believe the fundamental information we've covered in this book will set you up well to make the right choices for yourself, both now and long into the future. If I've done that, then I've accomplished my why. So, thank you for embarking upon this journey with me. And to that end, I wish you a long, healthy, and impactful life.

KEY TAKEAWAYS

1. **Technology enhances but won't replace the fundamentals.** Despite rapid technological advancement in areas like AI, nanobots, and brain-computer interfaces, the foundational pillars of exercise, nutrition, sleep, and stress management remain essential. The most effective approach to longevity integrates both technology and the timeless basics, all guided by your personal why that provides the motivation to make consistent healthy choices.

2. **Humans consistently underestimate the pace and impact of technological change.** Our linear thinking prevents us from accurately conceptualizing exponential technological growth. Technologies that seem like science fiction today may become commonplace within our lifetimes. Just as smartphones and the internet would have seemed impossible to previous generations, current technological developments will likely produce advancements we can't even imagine today.

3. **Wearable technology can provide useful data for crafting your own longevity framework.** Modern wearable devices track vital metrics and physical activity patterns that correlate strongly with longevity outcomes. These technologies can help you monitor trends and make adjustments to your lifestyle based on personalized data, rather than relying on generalized health advice.

You can find a list of all the specific interventions from this chapter in the Technology Cheat Sheet at TranscendHealthGroup.com/Resources.

CONCLUSION

We began this book with a simple question: Why do you want to live a longer, healthier life? The answer to that question—your why—has guided us through every chapter, from understanding the hallmarks of aging to implementing practical interventions that can add meaningful years to your life.

What we've discovered together is that longevity isn't about escaping death—it's about expanding life. It's about creating more moments of presence with those you love, more years of pursuing what matters most to you, and more opportunities to make the impact only you can. When you choose to live intentionally now, you're not just adding years to your life; you're adding life to your years.

The knowledge you now possess has given you the ability to reapproach and reexamine your health and the habits that surround it. If I've done my job right, you should now understand how the choices you make today directly influence the machinery that underlies your cellular aging. If I've really done a good job, you'll also know that AMPK and mTOR aren't just scientific acronyms but pathways you can modulate through intentional daily decisions, and how those interventions fit into your own life. All jokes aside, my hope is that even if you haven't retained all the nuanced details, you'll walk away from this book with a more informed outlook on how to preserve and maximize the functions of your incredible brain and body.

Perhaps the most empowering insight from our journey together is that your health outcomes are largely within your control. Outside of a handful of rare exceptions, the evidence clearly shows that maintaining healthy exercise, nutrition, and sleep habits will get you far. Managing stress, obtaining the right micronutrients through supplementation, incorporating hormetic stressors, and using technology to your maximum advantage can get you even further. The small choices you make each day compound over time, which means the best time to start is now, and that it's never too late. Make no doubt about it, you have the power to significantly influence your healthspan and lifespan right now.

Longevity isn't about perfection; it's about creating a sustainable approach that aligns with your life. The most effective exercise routine is the one you'll maintain. The optimal nutrition plan is the one you can follow consistently. The ideal sleep schedule works with your natural chronotype, not against it. In my view, the best way to approach your longevity is to craft a framework that reflects your preferences, your constraints, and most importantly, your purpose.

Imagine, for a moment, what that framework might feel like for you in the near future. Picture waking up every day knowing exactly what you need to do to keep your body healthy, your mind active, and make meaningful progress toward your why. Picture making the right choices not out of obligation, but because you're naturally inclined to do so. Now picture living that life, day in and day out, for decades to come. Imagine the impact your daily actions could have over a long, capable, fulfilling lifetime. This is all possible for you, and you're already well on your way there.

Before we part ways, I have a few things I feel compelled to share with you.

As I was working on this book, I sometimes received feedback that I was going into too much depth or that people didn't need to know every single detail I planned to cover. Believe it or not, I did tone back *much* of the information I had prepared based on that advice, but I purposefully chose to keep a lot of it here because I truly believe that knowledge will serve you well. I therefore hope you have enjoyed reading through what, at times, felt like endless rambling on my part, as I have never been accused of being short-winded.

Through the writing process, I also found myself once again fascinated by the inner workings of the human body, which is something I haven't experienced to this depth since my first exposure to them in medical school. In many ways, this book has rekindled my own relationship with the science I fell in love with so many years ago, and I hope that our time together has instilled a similar fascination in you.

If you do appreciate the science behind how your body works or if you're looking for more guidance in your own longevity journey, I would encourage you to consider becoming a part of our family. As the science of longevity continues to evolve, I will be doing my best to bring new evidence to light and educate as many people as I can on how to live a longer, healthier life, which is what I currently do through my company, Transcend Health.

I welcome you to join our community by visiting Transcend HealthGroup.com. Here, you can sign up for our newsletter to stay up to date on the latest longevity developments, connect with me on social media, and explore our memberships and courses that have been designed to support you on your ongoing journey. Most of these resources have been designed to supplement the information in this book, so just know that what you've read is only the beginning. There's still a wealth of information at your disposal, and more arrives everyday thanks to the dedicated laboratories and clinics around the world constantly advancing our understanding of these wondrously complex processes.

I'd also like to say that I'm ever-grateful you've allowed me to contribute to your why. By prioritizing your health, you've not only chosen to enhance your own life but to create positive change that extends well beyond yourself. Every single person who takes charge of their health is in a better position to influence their community and to inspire others to pursue their own path to vitality, further expanding opportunity and showing more people what is possible.

And finally, I'd like to thank you for contributing to my own why. I am on a mission to help people live longer, healthier, more impactful lives. By reading this book and taking control of your health, you've become part of that mission. My only ask is that you share this knowledge with others. Whether it's by gifting this book to a friend, lovingly informing a relative that it's not too late to start exercising, or educating your children on healthy nutritional habits, you are now armed with vital knowledge to benefit others. These small actions can create a ripple with the power to change the world.

That is the power you now hold. There's no greater love or virtue than living in the service of others. Together, we can elevate the collective health of our communities, our society, and the planet, and that is a why I believe we can all embrace.

Here's to your health, your purpose, and the extraordinary life that awaits.

With deep love and gratitude,
Ryan

ACKNOWLEDGMENTS

As I shared in the introduction, the motivation behind this book has been a lifetime in the making. I've always felt called to help more people, and this undertaking quickly became far more complex, humbling, and collaborative than anything I could have ever hoped to accomplish on my own.

With that in mind, I owe the completion and any success this book ultimately realizes to the array of amazing people who have dedicated their valuable time to me at all points in my life.

This list is by no means exhaustive and in that regard has made this the most challenging section to write. Countless people, experiences, and moments have shaped my perspective and contributed to my ultimate privilege of writing *The Incredible Brain*.

To all who have impacted my journey, whether briefly or from my first waking moments on earth, I offer my sincerest gratitude.

First and foremost, I want to thank every one of my patients—across all stages of my training and clinical practice. You have been my greatest teachers, constant motivators, and the very reason I continue to serve in this work.

To my mother, Margaret; my father, Alan; and my stepmother, Barbara—thank you for raising me with love, integrity, and for providing me with the best opportunity possible to live a life of meaning, for I have finally found it.

To all of my extended family, especially those who I have lost, your burden, while difficult to bear, has deep purpose—to help relieve suffering for others. Your strength and love are not forgotten and your legacy lives on:

To my grandmother Gog, whose unconditional love filled my early years with warmth.

To my grandfather Grumps, who, despite being trapped in a failing body, still radiated joy and humor.

To my aunt Charlotte, whose steadfast love introduced me early to the wonders of science and medicine and whose immutable courage showed me how to face disease with grace.

To my uncle Richard, who never let his illness define him nor dim his spirit or his wry smile—"Because you deserve what every individual should enjoy regularly."

To my grandmother Nannie, whose love, humor, and cooking were the foundation of our family.

And to my hero, my grandfather Papa—a true giant in every sense. Through our shared passions for medicine, motorsports, and the military, you gave me both shoulders to stand on and footsteps to follow.

You all remain alive within me, and in the hearts of those you touched. Your legacy helped inspire every word of this book.

To the professors who fueled my hunger for knowledge, in particular the late Dr. Charles Ouimet, Dr. Lynn Romrell, Dr. Robert Campbell, Dr. Christopher Leadem, Dr. Graham Patrick, Dr. John Blackmon, Dr. Jose Diaz, Dr. Gail Galasko, Dr. Lisa Granville, Dr. Alma Littles, Dr. Charles Maitland, Dr. Robert Watson, Dr. Bruce Berg, Dr. Ed Bradley, Dr. Nicole Bentze, Dr. Washington C. Hill, Dr. Richard Jamison, Dr. Sidney Holec, Dr. Kathleen Kennedy, Dr. Cynthia Samra, Dr. Jon Yenari, Dr. Dean Sutherland, Dr. Julio Cantero, Dr. Mauricio Concha, Dr. Kyle Ruffing, Dr. Arnoldo Perez-Singh, Dr. Martha Price, Dr. Fred Yturralde, Dr. Leonie Van Passel, and so many others.

ACKNOWLEDGMENTS

To Dean John Fogarty—thank you for believing in me and for setting the example of true leadership when it mattered most.

To the incredible physicians who shaped my clinical training: Dr. Carlo Tornatore, Dr. Laxman Bahroo, Dr. Robert Laureno, Dr. Carlos Mora, Dr. Gholam Motamedi, Dr. Jess Ailani, Dr. Carrie Dougherty, Dr. Fernando Pagan, Dr. Doug Mayson, Dr. Matthew Edwardson, Dr. Andy Stemer, Dr. Steven Lo, Dr. Faria Amjad, Dr. Fahd Amjad, Dr. Prerna Malla, Dr. Ishita Gambhir, Dr. Shakti Nayar, Dr. Benjamin Osborne, Dr. Robert Shin, Dr. Michael Sirdofsky, Dr. Francis Tirol, Dr. Tricia Ting, Dr. Peter Turkeltaub, Dr. Joseph Choi, Dr. Mark Lin—and many others.

To my brothers and sisters in the United States Navy and Marine Corps, and all our servicemembers past, present, and future—your courage, sacrifice, and camaraderie have inspired me more than you'll ever know. Serving alongside you remains one of the greatest honors of my life.

To Justin Donald and the Lifestyle Investor community—thank you for setting the bar for what it means to live with integrity, generosity, and purpose. Your selfless example has forever changed my life for the better.

To Amber Vilhauer and the entire NGNG team—especially Megan O'Malley, Alexis Snell, Jess Andrews, and Katrina Scarlett—thank you for transforming this vision into a reality. Without your expertise and guidance, this book would still be nothing more than a dream.

To the team at KN Literary Arts—in particular Kelly Notaras, Amy Hosford, Roger Copenhaver, and Sheryl Zajechowski—thank you for getting this project to the finish line in spite of the bumps along the road. What a learning experience this has been for all of us and a testament to teamwork, commitment, and graceful understanding.

To Nirmala Nataraj—your deep insight and thoughtful attention elevated this manuscript beyond what I ever imagined. I am endlessly grateful for the clarity and beauty you brought to these pages.

To Olivia Freeman and Wendy Brick at Transcend Health—thank you for being the operational backbone of our mission to help more people live longer, healthier, more impactful lives. As you know, this book is a direct extension of that important work.

To my book cohort—Tim and Jane O'Brien, Morgan Bendle, Janet DeMarin, and Mario Matavesco—your feedback, wisdom, and encouragement have had a profound impact on this book's final form. I am honored to walk alongside you and call you friends.

To Aidan DiPrima—I simply don't have the words. Without your brilliance, patience, and uncanny ability to channel my voice and distill complex information, this book would still be years away. There is not another soul on the planet who could stomach me talking about neuroscience and longevity for hours on end—and then transform it into something both approachable and useful. Beyond our work together, I've truly cherished our growing friendship and watching you personally implement these strategies in your own life has given me renewed belief in their power. I can't thank you enough.

To Dr. Arthur Frankel—you helped save my marriage and, more importantly, helped me discover my truest self. Your insight, compassion, and belief in me helped make this work possible. I am forever grateful for your permanent impact on my life.

To my brother, Tanner—your life, though tragically brief, was luminous. Your ability to make people feel seen, loved, and valued lives on in all of us. Your spirit is woven into every line of this work. Though I can no longer call you and talk for hours or come see you, I know you're aware of it, and you let me know with every rainbow, falcon, and drop of rain. Thank you for a lifetime of adventures, lessons, and the privilege of growing into manhood alongside you. Know that your girls are well cared for and your legacy lives on.

And to my wife, Kori. From the moment we met during my final month of medical school, I warned you life with me wouldn't be easy. I've certainly kept that promise. Through the exhaustion of residency, our time in the Navy, seven moves, enduring our constant weeks apart halfway across the country, every one of my "greatest" ideas, and now this book, you've remained the heart and strength of our family. Thank you for your boundless love and patience—especially during the recent months I spent writing with Boh and Jax sprawled across my lap. I can't wait to see where our next adventure takes us.

ABOUT THE AUTHOR

Dr. Ryan Williamson, M.D., is a board-certified neurologist, Navy veteran, and founder of Transcend Health—a platform blending neuroscience with high-performance living. After earning his medical degree from Florida State University and completing neurology training at Georgetown University Hospital, Dr. Williamson served as a Lieutenant Commander in the U.S. Navy. Today, he helps individuals and leaders overcome brain fog, improve memory, and optimize cognitive performance for a longer, healthier, more impactful life. Through Transcend Health, he offers expert-driven protocols, educational memberships, and private coaching. His book "The Incredible Brain" shares the science-backed strategies behind his mission: to help people take control of their brain health, unlock their full potential, and build a legacy that lasts.

ADDITIONAL RESOURCES

As much as I wanted to include every piece of information and every method of every intervention in these pages, I quickly realized there wasn't enough room to contain it all.

That's why I've created a resource page at:

www.TranscendHealthGroup.com/Resources.

The resource page includes additional information, exercises, and "cheat-sheets" for each of the intervention chapters that detail the most pertinent material from the chapter. These are available to you right now, or you can download them as you read. Either way, I hope they provide value on your longevity journey.

I will do my best to update these resources so you can find the most current, evidence-based information without waiting for the next edition of this book. If you're interested in staying up to date on the latest longevity information, sign up for our newsletter at www.TranscendHealthGroup.com.

To be clear: these are *supplementary* resources. The core principles, science, and interventions are all detailed right here in your hands (sometimes in excruciating detail). This book stands completely on its own as your guide to longevity.

www.ingramcontent.com/pod-product-compliance
Lightning Source LLC
Chambersburg PA
CBHW020531030426
42337CB00013B/805